Save Your Life

With Awesome Apple Cider Vinegar

Becoming pH Balanced In an Unbalanced World

Blythe Ayne, PhD

Save Your Life With Awesome
Apple Cider Vinegar
Becoming pH Balanced in an Unbalanced World
Blythe Ayne, Ph.D.

Emerson & Tilman, Publishers
129 Pendleton Way #55
Washougal, WA 98671

Book & cover design by Blythe Ayne
Text © Blythe Ayne
Graphics: Pixabay – *Thank You!*

Other books in the *How to Save Your Life* series:
Save Your Life with the Dynamic Duo: Vitamins D3 & K2
Save Your Life with the Phenomenal Lemon & Lime
Save Your Life with the Power of pH Balance
Save Your Life with the Elixir of Water
Save Your Life with Stupendous Spices

www.BlytheAyne.com

ebook ISBN: 978-1-957272-42-9
Paperback ISBN: 978-1-957272-43-6
Hardbound ISBN: 978-1-957272-44-3
Large Print ISBN: 978-1-957272-45-0
Audiobook ISBN: 978-1-957272-46-7

[1. HEALTH & FITNESS/Diet & Nutrition/Nutrition
2. HEALTH & FITNESS/Healing
3. HEALTH & FITNESS/Diseases/General]
BIC: FM
First Edition

Save Your Life

With Awesome Apple Cider Vinegar

Becoming pH Balanced In an Unbalanced World

Blythe Ayne, PhD

Poetry & Photography:
Home & the Surrounding Territory
Life Flows on the River of Love

Audiobooks:
Save Your Life With The Phenomenal Lemon
Save Your Life with Stupendous Spices
The Darling Undesirables
The Heart of Leo
The People in the Mirror

Blythe Ayne's paperback, large print, hardback books, ebooks, & audiobooks may be purchased wherever books are sold
and at: www.BlytheAyne.com

TABLE OF CONTENTS:

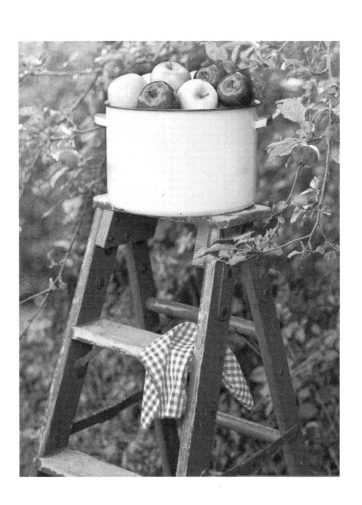

Chapter 1
A Bit of Info About Apple Cider Vinegar

"I stand in awe of my body."
Henry David Thoreau

A pple cider vinegar is antiseptic, antifungal, antiviral, antibacterial, antimicrobial, and anti-inflammatory, and has the power to kill ninety-eight percent of all germs.

Making Apple Cider Vinegar
First, the apples are chosen, then they're crushed. The juice is allowed to ferment via the yeasts in a container sealed tightly against exposure to oxygen.

Then there is a second fermentation when the apple cider is exposed to the air and bacteria, *acetobacter aceti*, which naturally occurs in the air, including enzymes and amino acids.

The Best Apple Cider Vinegar

Unfiltered, raw, apple cider vinegar is the best product to use. It's packed with vitamins, minerals, amino acids, magnesium, digestive enzymes, acetic acid, potassium, pectin, and polyphenols, which are natural antioxidants. The strands of visible proteins, enzymes, and bacteria, are known as "the Mother," which are the components largely responsible for its healing properties.

Filtered vinegar has gone through a process that eliminates the Mother, removing the majority of the efficacious and healing aspects of apple cider vinegar. Be sure to check that the product label says it contains "raw, unfiltered, apple cider vinegar, *with the Mother."*

The Benefits of Apple Cider Vinegar

Apple cider vinegar is rich in potassium, a mineral that is nearly universally lacking in the diets of Americans. Potassium requirements for the human body are two to five *grams* per day. That's grams. It's not easy to get this much potassium on a daily basis, and supplementation is generally advised.

Potassium is central to growth, building muscles, transmitting nerve impulses, and heart activity, along with preventing brittle teeth, hair loss, and runny noses.

These are just a few of its many wonders.

Apple cider vinegar is rich in acetic acid, which slows the digestion of starch and can help to lower the rise in glucose that commonly occurs after meals.

It's rich in malic acid, giving apple cider vinegar its antiviral, antibacterial, and antifungal properties, producing energy through the breakdown of fat calories. It also increases energy by dissolving toxins that cause fatigue and weakness, and it speeds up metabolism. Apple cider vinegar has health and life application from "soup to nuts."

Certain foods and deleterious habits, such as sugars, alcohol, simple carbs, artificial sugar, peanuts, most oils except olive and avocado, meat, dairy, and smoking, contribute to being overly acidic. Other foods, such as melons, dates, lemons, grapes, and apple cider vinegar, are alkaline and help balance the pH from the predominance of an acidic diet.

Over the centuries, vinegar has been used for many purposes: making pickles, killing weeds, polishing armor, as a disinfectant, a natural preservative, and making salads yummy. It has also been shown to kill cancer cells in numerous lab experiments.

Apple cider vinegar detoxifies and purifies. It breaks down fatty, mucous, phlegm deposits in the body, and, in doing so, improves the health and function of the kidneys, bladder, and liver.

It oxidizes the blood, reducing the risk of high blood pressure, and neutralizes toxic substances or harmful bacteria that enter the body when ingesting certain foods. Apple cider vinegar promotes healthy digestion, assimilation, and elimination.

Research has shown that apple cider vinegar assists in strengthening the heart, stabilizing blood sugar, and reducing the risk of a number of cancers. It flushes harmful toxins from the body and assists in weight control.

Apple Cider Vinegar Contents

According to the United States *National Institutes of Health* (NIH), and the *National Center for Biotechnology Information* (NCBI), apple cider vinegar contains the following:

"ACV consists of acetic acid, flavonoids such as gallic acid, tyrosol catechin, epicatechin, benzoic acid, vaninilin, caftaric acid, coutaric acid, caffeic acid, and ferrulic acid. These constituents have been reported to (positively) affect immune defense and oxidative responses.

"Apple cider vinegar is rich in calcium, chlorine, copper, iron, magnesium, phosphorous, potassium, silicon, sulfur, and other minerals in trace amounts. Apple cider vinegar is best known for its potassium content, which many people are deficient in, and is a powerful agent against high blood pressure. Apple cider vinegar is a source of Vitamin A, Vitamin B1, Vitamin B2, Vitamin B6, Vitamin C, Vitamin E, beta-carotene, and vitamin P. It is also rich in pectin."

There are several ongoing experiments discovering more acids and other elements in apple cider vinegar, which, to some extent, relates to the different apples, the different locations, and the different conditions—temperature, season, length of fermentation, and, literally the air from which the bacteria that manifests the apple cider vinegar, is created. A few of these not mentioned by the NIH are: malic acid, lactic acid, citric acid, succinic acid, chlorogenic acid, cis-p-coumaric acid, trans-p-coumaric acid, and phlorizin.

Apples, and thus apple cider vinegar, are high in procyanidins, which are more potent antioxidants than vitamins C or E, and have been shown to reduce LDL cholesterol. They also promote healthy blood vessels and are believed to contribute to longevity.

Apple cider vinegar also contains polyphenols. Polyphenols are naturally occurring organic compounds that have multiples of phenol units. Structurally diverse, they are found in abundance in plants.

Polyphenols Include
Flavonoids: Contain antioxidants. They reduce inflammation, interfere with cancer growth, and regulate essential enzyme functions.

Tannic Acid: A weak acid containing several phenol groups. It is used for chronic diarrhea, dysentery, bloody urine, painful joints, persistent coughs, and cancer, and is applied directly for bleeding. Tannic acid is also used in foods and beverages as a flavoring agent.

Ellagitannin: Ellagic acid is the product obtained from hydrolysis of ellagitannins. Ellagic acid is used for memory and thinking skills, to treat melasma—dark skin patches on the face, diabetes, and cancer, as well as many other purposes.

Polyphenols act as antioxidants in the body. Highly reactive oxygen molecules, known as free radicals, produced by external factors such as radiation, air pollution, smoking, chemical exposure, and, simply, normal cell processes, damage the body's healthy cells. Antioxidants to the rescue, which neutralize these free radicals.

And: *enzymes!*

It's all quite amazing!

Wikipedia lists the following components. Not that it's inaccurate, exactly, but it's a pale reflection of the actual complexity of apple cider vinegar with all its various, astounding, manifestations.

Per 100 Grams:

Energy (Calorie)	21kcal
Energy (joule)	90 kJ
carb	.93 g
sugar	.4g
Calcium	7 mg
Iron	.2 mg
Magnesium	5 mg
Phosphorus	8 mg
Potassium	73 mg
Sodium	5 mg
Zinc	.04 mg
Copper	.0008 mg
Manganese	.249 mg
Selenium	.1 iu
Water	93.81 grams

Below is a suggested dosage of apple cider vinegar. This standard suggested treatment is commonly noted throughout the many, many hundreds of references to apple cider vinegar I encountered in my research. But please keep in mind these guidelines are only a suggestion. You will learn for yourself what works best for you, or you and your health care professional, as you work together to manifest your best health.

Also, let me note that although I don't repeat the treatment for every entry in the book, you can refer back here to "Suggested Treatment."

Conversely, for those of you who read the book from cover to cover, please don't be frustrated by redundancies of information, but keep in mind that a book such as this is used as a reference, and therefore, treatment suggestions will be repeated intermittently for those who are looking for the specific information in their current particular case.

Apple Cider Vinegar is Acidic, But Burns in the Body as Alkalizing Ash

Certain foods, for example, apple cider vinegar and lemon, though acidic, leave an alkaline residue when burned to ash because of the type and amount of minerals they possess. Specifically, the calcium and potassium content of apple cider vinegar leaves an alkaline residue once burned, even though it was initially acidic.

Going a bit deeper into this rabbit hole, when apple cider vinegar is absorbed by the villi (the villi of the small intestine project into the intestinal cavity, increasing the surface area for food absorption and adding digestive secretions) into the blood, it goes to the liver. The liver sends the apple cider vinegar to be burned as fuel. Following that molecule in the energy cycle, when it's burned as energy, it leaves an alkalizing ash.

Additives

There is a veritable plethora of suggestions on how to use apple cider vinegar with additives; fruits, vegetables, oils, etc., etc., etc. I've not included them, (except for a couple of references to adding honey, and, of course, other ingredients in the recipe section), in the interest of making this book something that one can hold in two hands. If I were to include all of the literally *thousands* of ways that apple cider vinegar is and has been used, this book would become a ginormous tome.

But I do strongly encourage you to investigate for yourself what might be effective or tasty additives to your apple cider vinegar, once you've started using it, and have discovered its benefits. It can also be used in cooking, or sprinkled on salads and other vegetables. Drink it as a hot or cold beverage and sweeten it with honey.

Suggested Treatment

Mix from one teaspoon to two tablespoons of apple cider vinegar with eight ounces of water and drink it before each meal. Start with a teaspoon or two, and increase *gradually* to where you learn it's the most effective for you.

It's strongly recommended to dilute it in water or juice, as taking it straight will eventually harm the enamel on your teeth and perhaps your esophagus.

Apple cider vinegar is also extremely effective as a foot soak, or in the bath. A solution of one part apple cider vinegar to three parts water for the foot soak, or a cup in the bath, is effective.

Apple cider vinegar is often referred to as "ACV." However, I've chosen to write it out as a point of clarity, except when quoting a source that said "ACV".

Stating the somewhat obvious, your daily routine is healthiest when it also includes exercise, a well-balanced diet, and deep, rejuvenating *sl-e-e-e-e-p!*

*URLs for referred to studies can be found in **References and Resources**.

Chapter High Points:

1. The best apple cider vinegar is unfiltered, raw, and with the Mother. It's packed with vitamins, minerals, amino acids, magnesium, digestive enzymes, acetic and other acids, potassium, pectin, polyphenols, and other components, with an ever-growing list as experiments continue.

2. Apple cider vinegar is antiseptic, antifungal, antiviral, antibacterial, antimicrobial, and anti-inflammatory.

3. Apple cider vinegar detoxifies and purifies, oxidizes the blood, improves the function of the kidneys, bladder, and liver, strengthens the heart, stabilizes blood sugar, reduces the risk of a number of cancers, and assists in weight control. And the list goes on.

4. There are several suggested treatments, but the simplest is to drink one teaspoon to two tablespoons, according to taste and constitution, in a glass of water or juice, one to three times per day.

5. Apple cider vinegar is acidic, but burns in the body as alkalizing ash, helping to keep the blood slightly alkaline.

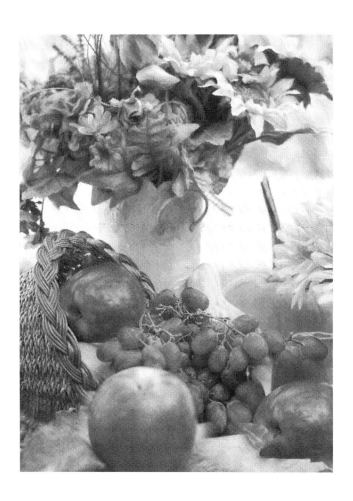

Chapter 2
Apple Cider Vinegar History

"A healthy attitude is contagious
but don't wait to catch it from others.
Be a carrier."
Tom Stoppard

A pples first appeared as a cultivated crop in Asia and Europe 8,000 years ago. And vinegar residues have been found in ancient Egyptian urns traced back to 3,000 BC, while the recorded history of vinegar in China dates back to 1,200 BC.

During biblical times, vinegar was used to flavor foods, as an energizing drink, and as a medicine. It is mentioned in both the old and new testaments several times.

In the Old Testament, after working a hard day gathering barley in the fields, Ruth was invited by Boaz to eat bread and dip it in vinegar. Ruth's timeline in history was probably between 1,160 BC and 1,100 BC. (Ruth 2:14)

This story of Ruth is reminiscent of Switchel, which you'll read about further on in the book. *Stay Tuned!*

In ancient Greece, around 400 BC, Hippocrates, the father of modern medicine, prescribed apple cider vinegar mixed with honey for a variety of ills including: coughs and colds, blood sugar reduction, decreasing cholesterol, increasing metabolism, speeding up weight loss, treating acid reflux and supporting gut health.

Hannibal crossed the Alps in 218 BC from Carthage to Italy by having his troops pour vinegar over boulders made hot by leaning trees against them and setting them on fire. The vinegar over the hot rocks caused them to fracture, and his troops were able to clear a path for his elephants.

Both Japanese samurai (646 AD, abolished in 1846) and Julius Caesar's army (60 BC) drank vinegar to boost their strength.

According to Pliny the Elder, the ancient Roman historian, Queen Cleopatra (Ruled 51-30 BC) taunted Marc Antony, saying that all his decadent feasts and displays of luxury were nothing compared to the lavishness she could exhibit.

She bet him she could spend 10,000,000 sesterces on one meal, roughly the equivalent of half-a-million dollars.

Marc Antony (he should have known better!) accepted the bet.

When Cleopatra had a sumptuous meal served, Marc Antony commented it was nothing spectacular. Then she called for the dessert course. Her servants placed a dish of vinegar in front of her. Cleopatra proceeded to take off one of her pearl earrings, which were known to be the largest pearls in the world at that time—and dropped it into the vinegar.

When the pearl dissolved, she drank it down. And won the bet.

Jumping ahead a few millennia to the 1300s, cider-making became quite popular in England. Many parishes paid their church tithes in hard cider, and the workers in monastery orchards were partially paid in cider. Two quarts a day for a man, and one quart a day for a boy.

In the middle of that same notable century, the black plague descended upon Europe and Asia. Thieves robbed the homes of the dead, wearing masks soaked in vinegar to protect them against the germs.

Christopher Columbus had vinegar on his ships to prevent scurvy.

Moving on to happier times, hard cider became currency in the American colonies. A parent recorded in a diary that he traded half-a-barrel of hard cider for his child's schooling. During this time, apple cider vinegar was even more valuable than hard cider, costing as much as three times more than hard cider.

A bleak moment in American history was during the temperance movement (1826), when activists took it upon themselves to chop down apple orchards to eradicate the ability to make hard apple cider. At the same time, it was served at temperance meetings, where they discussed ridding the United States of rum, whiskey, and other distilled alcohol.

Oh my goodness! Hypocrisy!

During the Civil War, soldiers sipped vinegar to prevent scurvy deficiency, and during both the Civil War (1861) and WWI (1914), vinegar was used to disinfect wounds.

Chapter High Points:

1. Apples have been cultivated for around 10,000 years, and vinegar residue in Egyptian urns as far back as 3000 BC.

2. Vinegar has been used for everything from healing diaper rash to killing cancer cells, to fracturing huge boulders, to allow for the passage of elephants.

3. Apple cider vinegar is the first electrolyte beverage, used by field workers for centuries, until the present day.

Note: apple cider vinegar may interact with certain drugs. If you take any of the following medications, please talk with your health care provider before beginning a regime of apple cider vinegar: Digoxin, insulin, diabetes drugs, diuretics, or water pills.

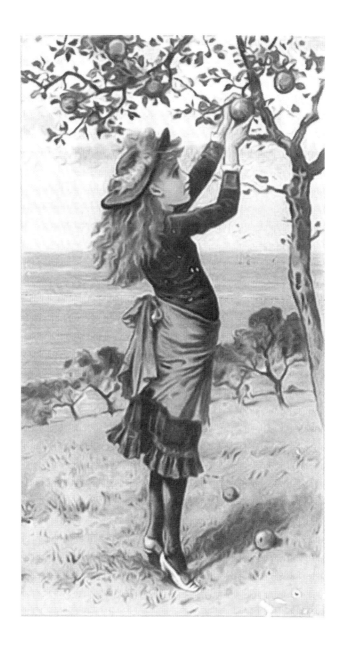

Chapter 3

Apple Cider Vinegar for the Body

"The body is a sacred garment."
Martha Graham

L et's dive into the absolutely *stunning* plethora of potential benefits humble-yet-healthy apple cider vinegar offers.

Apple Cider Vinegar for Aging
There are four main causes of aging:
• Formation of free radicals
• Decrease of energy production in the cell
• Degeneration of the cell membrane
• Changes in hereditary material

In short, aging is caused by changes in the cells over time, influenced, as well, by external factors. Stress and poor nutrition contribute to premature aging. *But!* There are also natural ways to preserve your youth and good health for many years.

Apple cider vinegar applied topically improves the epidermis, which assists cell regeneration. These antioxidant virtues allow apple cider vinegar to fight against free radicals, slowing down the aging process. When taken internally, apple cider vinegar helps rejuvenate the whole body! It's effective against joint pain, digestive problems, and weight gain.

Apple Cider Vinegar Stands up to Wrinkles
Whether addressing current wrinkles or preventing future ones, apple cider vinegar tones the skin, regaining elasticity and keeping it soft and silky.

Apply apple cider vinegar to the face diluted with water. Leave it on for about ten minutes, then rinse it off. For this routine to be effective, it needs to be done at least twice a week.

Apple Cider Vinegar for Both Dark and Light Skin Spots
Apple cider vinegar gets rid of dark spots, as well as those related to depigmentation. Apply apple cider vinegar to the affected areas and leave it on for as long as twenty minutes. Then rinse and dry. Do this regularly to see the skin rejuvenated. Apple cider vinegar, which contains alpha-hydroxy acids, removes dead skin and brightens it.

Adding a cup of apple cider vinegar to the bath water and soaking for twenty minutes or more is another way to let it work on your skin. The apple cider vinegar will rid the skin of toxins.

Apple Cider Vinegar for Allergies, Hives, & Impetigo

An allergic reaction that manifests as red, itchy bumps, urticaria, or hives, may be temporary or chronic, and may be responding to histamine, a chemical the body releases that makes blood vessels leak into the deep layers of the skin.

Anything that triggers an allergic reaction; pollen, dust, dander, dust mites, shellfish, etc., can cause hives. Hives can also manifest from excessive heat or cold, exposure to sunlight, and stress.

Apple Cider Vinegar's Anti-Inflammatory, Antihistamine Properties

Apple cider vinegar is effective in treating allergies and other skin issues because of its anti-inflammatory properties. It reduces itching and keeps swelling and redness in control. Its antihistamine properties regulate the body's immune response, limiting irritation and pain.

Add two cups apple cider vinegar to bath water and soak in it for fifteen to twenty minutes. Or wash the affected area with one-to-one apple cider vinegar and water two or three times a day.

Itchy mosquito bites are relieved by topical application of apple cider vinegar because it balances the pH of the skin. Many toxic substances become less toxic as apple cider vinegar changes toxins into a less toxic acetate compound—an excellent neutralizing agent for insect bites and skin allergies.

Impetigo

Impetigo is a contagious superficial bacterial infection that enters through lesions or cuts. It's most common among preschool and school-age children and is characterized by blisters or red sores. There are two forms, bullous and non-bullous. Non-bullous impetigo is more contagious than bullous.

Bullous impetigo is characterized by fragile blisters that break easily and appear without prior trauma to the skin. It may also cause fever, diarrhea, and fatigue. Non-bullous impetigo is characterized by small blisters with yellow crusts and is more common than bullous impetigo.

Impetigo is a highly contagious disease, spread by direct contact through sores or nasal discharge. Somewhat obviously, engaging in close-contact sports increases the risk of contracting impetigo. Pre-existing eczema, insect bites, burns, poison ivy, chemicals, and warm and humid temperatures can give impetigo a means of entry.

A suggested application is one-fourth cup of apple cider vinegar to two cups of water to clean the affected sores, which helps to remove and heal the scabs.

Apple Cider Vinegar for Anti-Cancer Properties

Many of the claims about apple cider vinegar and cancer originated from the work of scientist and Nobel Prize winner Otto Warburg. Dr. Warburg believed that cancer was a nutritional problem, and claimed that eighty percent of cancer cases were avoidable with a healthy, natural, pH-balanced, diet.

Warburg also suggested that high levels of acidity and low levels of oxygen in the body caused cancer. He based this hypothesis on the fact that cancer cells produce acid as they grow, even in environments that are not usually acidic.

Tumor Cells Die on Exposure to Acetic Acid

"Acetic acid promptly induced the cell death of (cancer cells). Acetic acid is a powerful anti-cancer agent. Topical application of acetic acid may be a feasible approach for the treatments of gastric cancer and possibly other malignancies."

Acetic Acid Induces Cell Death – https://onlinelibrary.wiley.com/doi/full/10.1111/jgh.12775

Apple cider vinegar's antioxidants help keep the body healthy and strong, able to fight cell-damaging free radicals.

Properties of Vinegar

"Therapeutic effects of vinegar arise from consuming the inherent bioactive components including acetic acid, gallic acid, catechin, ephicatechin, chlorogenic acid, caffeic acid, p-coumaric acid, and ferulic acid cause antioxidative, antidiabetic, antimicrobial, antitumor, anti-obesity, antihypertensive, and cholesterol-lowering responses."

Functional Properties of Vinegar – https://ift.onlinelibrary.wiley.com/doi/full/10.1111/1750-3841.12434

Anti-cancer Activities of Pectin

In 1825, French chemist and pharmacist, Henri Braconnot, an expert in extracting active components from plants, was the first to discover a heteropolysaccharide with gelling properties which he named "pectic acid."

Pectin is a natural prebiotic and increases butyrate, although its exact chemical structure is still not clear. Pectins are a family of acid-rich polymers. Three main pectic polysaccharides have been isolated from plant walls.

Researcher, Dr. F. Brouns notes, "Alternative practitioners often tout apple pectin as a cancer fighter. That's because it can bind to an intestinal enzyme called beta-glucuronidase. The enzyme comes from fecal bacteria. It's closely associated with colon cancer. A review of test-tube studies confirmed apple pectin could suppress beta-glu-curonidase in test-tube studies, and animal studies also suggest a benefit.

"Pectin displays properties useful in medicine. In humans, pectin, as a dietary fiber, is not enzymatically digested in the small intestine but is degraded by microbial in the colon. It keeps its gelling action in the digestive track, so that it slows down digestion. This is very beneficial in patients who have a too rapid digestion in their stomach.

"Pectin is also capable of diminishing blood cholesterol level, and stimulating lipid excretion.

"When colon adenocarcinoma cells were incubated in the presence of pectin oligosaccharides for three days, an increase in apoptosis (cell death) in DNA fragmentation was observed. *This is also true for cells from other types of cancer.* DNA fragmentation was directly proportional to the number of apoptotic cells.

"Colonocyte apoptosis activation in animals fed with pectin is also largely due to butyrate, a molecule coming from pectin fermentation by colon bacteria flora."

Pectin has been known for its anti-tumor activities for decades, playing a significant role in preventing colon cancer. As long ago as 1979, Dr. Watanabe and team demonstrated that rats treated with carcinogenic and neurotoxic chemical compounds developed fewer colon tumors if their diet was enriched with pectin.

Apple Cider Vinegar for Arthritis, Rheumatoid Arthritis, & Osteoarthritis

Probably the single most important aspect of apple cider vinegar when it comes to "The Itises" is the anti-inflammatory property of acetic acid, critical in improving joint pains. Also, apple cider vinegar's potassium proves its strength in helping to remove arthritis calcium deposits.

There are over one hundred different types of arthritis that have been identified. The two most common types are:

Osteoarthritis (OA)

Characterized by chronic inflammation of the joints.

Rheumatoid arthritis (RA)

Classified as an autoimmune disease, RA causes inflammation, predominantly affecting the joints in the body. Apple cider vinegar's pain-relieving abilities are due to its high acetic acid content, which helps negate excessive acidity in the blood that leads to inflammation and thus, *pain*. Again, although apple cider vinegar contains acetic acid, once it is metabolized in the body, it becomes alkaline.

Apple cider vinegar is also rich in antioxidants, which help prevent damage from free radicals that contribute to stiff, painful joints.

Apple Cider Vinegar and Osteoarthritis
Apple cider vinegar poultices and soaks can be effective for pain management, along with internal use. Consuming apple cider vinegar helps balance the body's pH levels, reducing acid buildup that contributes to severe joint pain.

Apple Cider Vinegar & Rheumatoid Arthritis
Apple cider vinegar can help dissolve crystals that build up in the joints of people suffering from rheumatoid arthritis, eliminating the crystals from the body through the kidneys and bladder.

Apple Cider Vinegar and Arthritis—the Research
Dr. Deforest Clinton Jarvis published his findings regarding apple cider vinegar in his book, *Folk Medicine*. He stated that "Numerous common ailments including … rheumatism and arthritis may be relieved, and even cured with this simple (apple cider vinegar) treatment."

A study conducted by the *Mashhad University of Medical Sciences* found that apple cider vinegar was effective at reducing chronic inflammation and pain in arthritis sufferers. The benefits were thought, in part, to be due to the complex of B vitamins in apple cider vinegar.

In addition to taking your daily dose of apple cider vinegar and water, soak the arthritic joint in a warm-to-hot, strong solution of half-a-cup of apple cider vinegar to three cups of water. If not practical or not comfortably accessible to soak the area, soak cheesecloth or a washcloth in the vinegar and water solution, wrap it around the area, then wrap it in cling wrap to keep the heat in. This procedure may be repeated as often as you like.

Apple Cider Vinegar for Asthma & Bronchitis

Bronchitis is a condition of the lining of the bronchial tubes becoming inflamed, resulting in coughing, chest discomfort, fever, and fatigue. Apple cider vinegar is a natural remedy for these conditions because it lowers inflammation in the lungs and stops the growth of bacteria and viruses.

Apple cider vinegar's acetic acid has antimicrobial and anti-inflammatory properties, as well as nutrients from the apples. A *Scientific Reports* study noted that apple cider vinegar not only halted the growth of various microbial species, including *E. coli* and *S. aureus*, but also helped prevent the release of pro-inflammatory cytokines, a protein that triggers inflammation.

Apple cider vinegar can also ease asthma symptoms by reducing esophageal reflux when the contents of the stomach back up into the esophagus and irritate the airways. Other symptoms of GERD include asthma-like hoarseness and chronic cough.

A suggested remedy is to stir one tablespoon of apple cider vinegar into a glass of water and sip over the next half hour to subside wheezing. This is diluted enough that it is unlikely to damage tooth enamel, but it's not a bad idea to drink straight water, as well.

Another treatment that many people have reported works well is to soak a cloth in apple cider vinegar and apply to wrists with pressure.

According to the *Cleveland Clinic Foundation*, "It is esti-mated that more than seventy-five percent of patients with asthma also experience gastroesophageal reflux disease (GERD). People with asthma are twice as likely to have GERD as those who do not."

The acidity in apple cider vinegar helps the hydrochlo-ric acid of the stomach do its job, a contributing factor in why apple cider vinegar relieves both acid reflux *and* asthma.

Apple Cider Vinegar for Athletes' Foot
Athletes' foot is a fungal infection that usually develops when wearing damp socks and shoes, or engaging in sporting activities in hot and humid conditions. An effec-

tive remedy is apple cider vinegar. It will clear the fungal infection that causes athletes' foot, and at the same time reduce pain and inflammation caused by the condition.

Soak your feet in a fifty-fifty solution of apple cider vinegar for thirty minutes. There is likely to be a burning sensation, but as long as you can tolerate it, it is healing. If it is not tolerable, dilute with more water. Continue this treatment on a daily basis until the fungal infection is gone.

Apple cider vinegar also treats foot odor by balancing the pH level of your feet.

Apple Cider Vinegar for Autoimmune Disease

Seventy to eighty percent of your immune system lives in the gut. Apple cider vinegar supports healthy bacterial balance in the gut, contributing to a stronger, more efficient immune system.

A healthy gut helps the immune system in the following ways:
• Prevents illness or infection
• Supports the body's healing response to infection
• Aids in a faster recovery time

Research confirms that the probiotics in apple cider vinegar support a strong immune response. Participants who received probiotics in a study that examined the effects on upper respiratory illness and flu-like symptoms had statistically significant health improvements when compared to the placebo group. The probiotics addressed cough, nasal congestion, headache, muscle pain, and other flu-like symptoms.

When it comes to optimizing the body's immune function, apple cider vinegar works wonders. By promoting a healthy gut microbiome, this ancient remedy strengthens the immune response and leads to improvements in overall health.

Apple Cider Vinegar for Bleeding

For nose bleeds, put a few drops of apple cider vinegar on a cotton pad and apply it in your nostrils, which will lower the blood flow.

Excessive Shedding of the Uterine Wall

Any changes in the levels of estrogen and progesterone can lead to the excessive shedding of the uterine wall. Obesity, diabetes, thyroid disorder, and polycystic ovarian syndrome (PCOS) can cause hormonal imbalance.

If the ovaries don't release an egg during the menstrual cycle, it can cause heavy bleeding, which can also develop as a side effect of using a non-hormonal IUD.

Noncancerous uterine fibroids or benign polyp-like growths can sometimes be the reason for heavy or prolonged menstrual cycles, while prolonged bleeding with severe fatigue and cramps in postmenopausal women can be an indication of cervical or uterine cancer.

In addition, blood-thinning medications and anti-inflammatory drugs can cause prolonged cycles.

Effect Of Apple Cider Vinegar
A scientific study found that regular consumption of apple cider vinegar can boost fertility and make periods regular.

Hemorrhoids
Hemorrhoids can be internal or external. When an internal hemorrhoid prolapses (bulges outward) it can bring with it mucus that can aggravate the irritation and cause itching.

Apple cider vinegar's acetic acid is astringent, which shrinks organic tissues. It also has antibacterial and anti-fungal properties. It suppresses inflammation and provides relief from pain and itching.

If applying externally, diluting apple cider vinegar with water can reduce the risk of skin irritation, while providing relief. Taken internally, over time its astringent and antiseptic qualities will help improve the condition.

Apple Cider Vinegar and the Brain

The benefits of apple cider vinegar for the brain are numerous. It has anti-inflammatory, anti-depressant, anti-anxiety, antioxidant, and cognitive-boosting properties. It contains probiotic properties, stimulating good bacteria.

Apple cider vinegar taken before meals helps proteins break down into amino acids, which leads to the formation of tryptophan, which plays a significant role in releasing the "feel good" neurotransmitter, serotonin, elevating mood, and letting you feel happy and relaxed.

A study published by the *American Chemical Institute* observed that apple cider vinegar can improve cognitive function and slow dementia.

Arizona State University researchers investigated the role of apple cider vinegar in mental health, given its gut-brain connection. Their study consisted of twenty-five healthy college students. For four weeks, half of the students were given a placebo and the other half were given apple cider vinegar.

Significant Reduction in Depression

The study showed that the subjects who consumed apple cider vinegar experienced a twenty to thirty-four percent reduction in depressive mood. Somewhat surprisingly, those who were given the placebo registered a slight increase in depression. Apple cider vinegar positively affects metabolic pathways of the brain. It promotes a healthier hexosamine pathway (simple sugars that have six carbon atoms per molecule) that encourages strong cognitive functioning and brain health.

Additionally, drinking apple cider vinegar improves glycine and threonine metabolism, amino acids that balance neurotransmitters, and stimulate hormones like serotonin.

A study titled: *Daily Vinegar Ingestion Improves Depression Scores and Alters the Metabolome in Healthy Adults: A Randomized Controlled Trial* had the following results:

There were clear distinctions between subject and placebo groups. Several of the metabolic alterations associated with vinegar ingestion were consistent for improved mood, including significant increases in glycine, serine, and threonine metabolism. Acetic acid is the major ingredient in vinegar, and ingestion results in a rapid rise in serum acetate.

Another report demonstrated that the depletion of acetate-producing bacteria in the gut microbiota in a rat study of type 1 diabetes accelerated cognitive decline. This decline was reversed by oral acetate (apple cider vinegar) supplementation.

Apple cider vinegar improves gut health. When the gut is off-balance, it interferes with mental health and general well-being.

Apple Cider Vinegar for Colds, Flu, Fever & Sore Throat

There are almost two hundred types of viruses that cause colds. The virus attaches itself to the mucous membranes of the nose and throat, forcing cells to replicate more virus cells. Coughing, sneezing, fatigue, itchy eyes, fever, and congestion are caused when the body's defense system is working to fight off the virus and boost the immune system.

Being infected with a cold can lead to complications such as pneumonia, acute bronchitis, strep throat, and acute bacterial sinusitis. Apple cider vinegar alkalizes the body, making it difficult for the cold virus to get a footing in the first place, or if it does, to continue.

Apple cider vinegar's potassium helps thin mucus, and its acetic acid inhibits bacterial growth that contributes to congestion of the nasal passages. It has antimicrobial and antioxidant properties that kill bacteria, yeasts, and fungal infections. Its polyphenolic compounds are antioxidants that prevent the formation of tissue-damaging free radicals.

The Mother in apple cider vinegar, which is yeast and bacteria, is immune-boosting probiotics, fighting flu respiratory infections.

Gargling with apple cider vinegar kills germs, eases a sore throat, and prevents the development of a more severe condition, such as strep throat. Apple cider vinegar is rich in antibacterial properties that heal bacterial infections in the throat.

Add a couple of tablespoons of apple cider vinegar to a vaporizer to relieve cold, flu, sinus, and chest infections.

Apple Cider Vinegar for Constipation & Diarrhea

The most common causes of constipation include: lack of exercise, not enough liquids, not enough fiber in the diet, medications, changes in habits or lifestyle, travel, pregnancy, and/or overuse of laxatives. Though occasional constipation is common, some people experience chronic constipation that can interfere with their ability to go about their daily lives.

Diarrhea can be due to bacterial or viral infections, consumption of contaminated water or food, or food intolerances, among possible other causes. The result is frequent evacuation of the bowels, due to inflammation and irritation of the mucous membrane of the intestines.

Apple cider vinegar is a bacteria, virus, parasite, and microbe destroyer, eliminating *E. coli* bacteria and clearing the symptoms associated with diarrhea and constipation, such as stomach ache, nausea, and intestinal spasms. It maintains proper pH levels in the stomach, allowing the growth of good bacteria. It replenishes the body's potassium and magnesium. It acts as a natural laxative for constipation.

Apple cider vinegar contains pectin, adding water-soluble fiber to the diet, which improves overall digestion and eliminates harmful toxins. Pectin also forms a protective layer to soothe the irritated lining of the colon. It swells up, and the bulk eases diarrhea. Taking apple cider vinegar before a meal can even *prevent* diarrhea.

Apple cider vinegar's acetic acid and malic acid help in digestion and detoxification, while defending against viruses, bacteria, and fungi.

Begin the standard apple cider vinegar protocol cautiously with one teaspoon to two tablespoons in a glass of water, one to three times per day, and continue one or two days after the problem has resolved.

Or continue apple cider vinegar as a daily habit, which is probably the wisest choice of all!

Apple Cider Vinegar for Chicken Pox & Shingles

Chickenpox is a highly contagious disease caused by the varicella-zoster virus (VZV). It causes an itchy, blister-like rash. The rash first appears on the chest, back, and face, and then spreads over the entire body in hundreds of itchy blisters.

Shingles, also caused by the zoster virus, is a painful, blistery rash. Older adults or people with illnesses that weaken their immune systems are more susceptible to shingles. The virus can strike at any time, affecting a different part of the body.

Apple cider vinegar is an effective remedy that will help expedite a rapid recovery and can be used orally or topically. It has antiviral, anti-inflammatory, and antimicrobial properties, a perfect combination for treating and soothing chickenpox and shingles. Drinking apple cider vinegar promotes healing, and using it topically reduces inflammation.

Dilute one tablespoon of apple cider vinegar in a cup of water and apply it to the blisters or rash. The acidity of apple cider vinegar eases the itching, helps dry the blisters, and suppresses the virus. It will sting the open blisters, but if tolerated, it does help them to heal, and ultimately reduces the pain.

Or take a bath with apple cider vinegar added. Run a warm bath and add a cup of apple cider vinegar. Soak for twenty to thirty minutes to soothe the rash and promote healing. Repeat daily until healed.

Apple cider vinegar has many antimicrobial properties and will give instant relief from itching. It reduces scarring and heals lesions before they develop.

Apple Cider Vinegar for Cholesterol
Cholesterol is found in much of our food, and the body produces it as well. It is required by the body to produce steroidal hormones, including progesterone and testosterone. It's also essential to synthesize vitamin D and bile acids that aid in digestion. The problem occurs when there's an excess of LDL cholesterol, clogging arteries and restricting blood flow.

Cholesterol binds to protein receptors in the bloodstream and travels around the body, forming lipoproteins. The proportion of protein to lipids determines each of the two types of cholesterol.

The Difference Between LDL & HDL

High-density lipoproteins (HDL), the good type, contain *more* protein than cholesterol. Low-density lipoproteins (LDL), contain *less* protein than cholesterol.

The reason LDL cholesterol is problematic is that the excessive cholesterol oxidizes in the bloodstream, forming thick, hard, plaque deposits that clog arteries. Eventually, this becomes atherosclerosis, with its attending blood clots and high blood pressure. Atherosclerosis in the coronary arteries leads to an increased probability of stroke or heart attack.

Enter the guys in the white hats, the HDLs, who round up and transport the LDL deposits and shunt them to the liver. The liver's job is to flush them out of the body.

But! When there are more LDLs than the HDLs can handle, and add to the battle those fat triglycerides, the body simply becomes vulnerable to a number of diseases.

Good News!
Here's the good news … there have been many studies that show that consuming apple cider vinegar can help reduce bad cholesterol levels. One study featured normal and diabetic rats. The low-density lipoproteins were reduced and the high-density lipoproteins were increased in the normal rats taking apple cider vinegar. With the diabetic rats, apple cider vinegar reduced the levels of triglycerides, while increasing the

number of high-density lipoproteins. Not only a win for the diabetic rats but also a notable win for the healthy rats!

Another study, featuring rabbits, had a similar conclusion, with apple cider vinegar reducing atherosclerosis in the group that had a high-cholesterol diet.

Apple Cider Vinegar Fights Oxidative Stress
Oxidative stress, due to free radical damage, is a significant factor in the onset and progression of atherosclerosis. Another study showed that apple cider vinegar scavenges free radicals, preventing oxidative stress, and increasing the number of antioxidant enzymes and vitamins.

Apple Cider Vinegar Reduces LDL Oxidation
Apple cider vinegar's anti-oxidative attributes come from its flavonoids; quercetin, catechin, phloridzin, and chlorogenic acid. Taking these polyphenolic natural antioxidants inhibits the oxidation of low-density lipoproteins.

Apple Pectin Lowers LDL
The apple pectin in apple cider vinegar is a soluble fiber. Its main component is galacturonic acid, a type of sugar acid that binds to bile in the intestines. Digestive enzymes can't break down pectin, but gut bacteria can and does.

Apple pectin also helps lower cholesterol. In one study specifically focusing on pectin, it lowered LDL cholesterol between seven and ten percent.

Apple Cider Vinegar for Depression

Depression is becoming ever-more prevalent, with more and more people seeking help. Apple cider vinegar has natural mood boosters that help increase blood sugar levels by assisting in the digestion process, as they break down the enzymes in the stomach and intestines. It can do away with that tired feeling when depressed, providing an extra boost. A sense of strength is regained, both mentally and physically.

Apple cider vinegar, when taken before meals, helps the proteins in food be broken down into amino acids, which leads to the creation of tryptophan, which, as previously mentioned, plays a critical role in releasing the "feel good" neurotransmitter, serotonin.

Apple cider vinegar also has an impact on weight loss. A loss in weight leads to lower cholesterol levels and, again, higher tryptophan creation. So, on days when depression is keeping your brain from making serotonin, apple cider vinegar can give it some help.

Another plus is that apple cider vinegar doesn't have to be taken every day to work because it doesn't need to build up in the system, as is the case with antidepressants. You can decide how and when you want to take it, depending on how you're feeling.

Apple Cider Vinegar for Diabetes
The effect of apple cider vinegar on blood sugar levels is among the most intensely researched—and most promising!—of apple cider vinegar's potential health benefits. A compelling application of apple cider vinegar is helping treat type 2 diabetes, characterized by high blood sugar levels caused by insulin resistance, or the inability to produce insulin.

"Diabetes mellitus (DM) was first recognized as a disease around 3,000 years ago by the ancient Egyptians and East Indians, illustrating clinical features similar to what we now know as diabetes. Poorly controlled diabetes can damage various organs, especially the eyes, kidneys, nerves, and cardiovascular system."

Effect of Diet on Type 2 Diabetes Mellitus – https:// www.ncbi.nlm.nih.gov/pmc/articles/PMC5426415/

Apple cider vinegar has shown great promise in improving insulin sensitivity and helping lower blood sugar responses after meals.

Apple Cider Vinegar Lowers Glucose

Insulin-resistant participants in a study titled: "*Vinegar Improves Insulin Sensitivity to a High Carbohydrate Meal in Subjects with Insulin Resistance on Type Two Diabetes*," were given apple cider vinegar before a high carbohydrate snack of orange juice and a bagel. Apple cider vinegar lowered the glucose of the insulin-resistant participants, by as much as thirty-four percent, and insulin spikes were significantly reduced!

A study titled, "*Examination of the Anti-glycemic Properties of Vinegar in Healthy Adults*," investigated the effect of two different doses of apple cider vinegar. Interestingly, it was found that ten grams (approximately two teaspoons) were just as effective as twenty grams. Also, taking the vinegar just before the meal was more effective than taking it five hours before the meal.

Type 2 diabetics, who were not on insulin, were the participants in the study titled, "*Vinegar Ingestion at Bedtime Moderates Waking Glucose Concentrations*." They were given two tablespoons of apple cider vinegar at bedtime. There was a measurable effect in lowering their morning blood sugars, although the effect was small.

Numerous other laboratory studies with humans show that vinegar can improve insulin function and lower blood sugar levels after meals.

High Blood Sugar Levels Contribute to A Variety of Chronic Diseases

Furthermore, people *without* diabetes can also benefit from keeping their blood sugar levels in the normal range, as there is compelling evidence that high blood sugar levels are a significant contributor to a variety of chronic diseases and aging.

Bear in mind that people who have elevated blood glucose levels have a greater chance of developing type 2 diabetes. Acetic acid in raw apple cider vinegar helps balance blood sugar levels and enhances insulin response and insulin sensitivity.

In summation, taking one to two tablespoons of apple cider vinegar that contains the Mother in a glass of water before meals has been shown to reduce the risk of developing type 2 diabetes.

Discuss using apple cider vinegar with your healthcare practitioner if you are taking diabetes medication or diuretic drugs, as apple cider vinegar may cause hypoglycemia or hypokalemia—low potassium. Because apple cider vinegar slows digestion (very good in most instances), it can contribute to lowering potassium levels in conjunction with the diabetes medication, even more (not good in these cases).

Apple Cider Vinegar for Ear Infections & Tinnitus

Tinnitus, the term used to describe ringing in one or both ears, affects about ten to fifteen percent of the population. Infections of the outer ear or middle ear can lead to tinnitus. These infections are caused by bacteria such as *E. Coli* and *Staphylococcus aureus*.

Even in low doses, apple cider vinegar has antibacterial properties, inhibiting the growth of bacteria and reducing inflammation. In higher concentrations, apple cider vinegar can destroy the bacteria's cell wall, wiping out the damaging bacteria, and by extension, helping to control the prominent factors causing tinnitus.

Symptoms

Tinnitus usually has a very gradual onset, becoming worse until it is loud and distracting. The symptoms of tinnitus are commonly described as ringing in the ears, but it has also been described as humming, hissing, buzzing, roaring, screeching, or whooshing. There may be periods when the sound abates, or it may be non-stop.

The following are typical causes of tinnitus:

Hearing Loss

The sensory organ responsible for hearing is the cochlea. Sound waves are detected by tiny hairs that stimulate nerve impulses. Unfortunately, however, the cochlea hairs wear out over time. The gradual wearing away, breaking, or bending of these hairs manifests as a loss of hearing, or even inaccurate signals to the brain, interpreted as sound.

Canal Blockage
The ear canal may become blocked by fluid, earwax, debris, or dirt, resulting in pressure changes that may cause tinnitus.

Infection
Bacteria or virus can cause an ear infection in the outer ear (Otitis Externa) and/or the middle ear (Otitis Media) manifesting as inflammation, fluid buildup, irritation, pain, and tinnitus. Antibiotics may be used to treat an ear infection, and when successful, the tinnitus generally disappears.

Medications
Diuretics, antibiotics, antidepressants, NSAIDs, and cancer drugs are all implicated in causing or aggravating tinnitus.

Head or Neck Injuries
Partial or even total hearing loss may be the result of a head or neck injury that affects the cranial nerves connected to hearing, causing tinnitus as well, which generally only occurs in one ear.

Tinnitus may also be caused by head or neck tumors, eustachian tube dysfunctions, acoustic neuromas,

Meniere's disease, ear bone disorders, blood vessel disorders, as well as other diseases and dysfunctions.

Apple Cider Vinegar Aids Tinnitus
Because of its antibacterial qualities, apple cider vinegar can alleviate bacterial infections, including tinnitus. It kills bacteria like *Staphylococcus aureus* and *E. Coli,* known to cause ear infections.

Apple cider vinegar can be used in a variety of ways to treat ear infections or tinnitus.

Apple Cider Vinegar Ear Drops
Mix an equal amount of apple cider vinegar with lukewarm water. Apply five to ten drops in the affected ear canal, holding the head sideways. Hold this position for around five minutes. Then tilt your head in the opposite direction to drain, and repeat in the other ear.

Gargling with Apple Cider Vinegar
Gargling with apple cider vinegar and warm water can help heal an eustachian tube infection. As the ear and the throat have a close relationship, gargling with apple cider vinegar can be very effective. Again, mix an equal amount of warm water and apple cider vinegar, then gargle for thirty seconds. Repeat two or three times daily.

Apple Cider Vinegar for Eyes
The anthocyanin in apple cider vinegar called cyanidin is a flavonoid phytochemical and an antioxidant that improves vision and healthy eyes.

Apple Cider Vinegar for Itchy Eyes
Whether your eyes are feeling itchy from a cold, flu, allergies, or simply being tired, a couple doses a day of apple cider vinegar with its anti-inflammatory and antihistamine properties will help calm the itching.

Dark Circles under the Eyes
Pat a little apple cider vinegar on the dark circles under the eyes morning and evening. It will brighten the skin under your eyes in a few days. Be sure not to get undiluted apple cider vinegar in your eyes.

Apple Cider Vinegar for Cataracts
A cataract is a cloudy area in the lens of the eye. Over half of all Americans over the age of eighty either have cataracts, or have had surgery to get rid of them. Over time, cataracts can make vision blurry, hazy, and less clear. Cataracts cause approximately fifty percent of blindness in the world. Apple cider vinegar's antioxidant properties help prevent cataracts. A couple of doses a day contributes to clear vision.

Apple Cider Vinegar for Fibromyalgia, CFS, & Adrenal Fatigue

Fibromyalgia, chronic fatigue, and adrenal fatigue have their differences, but they also have a few similarities. Here's some information about each syndrome, and what apple cider vinegar can do to help alleviate the symptoms.

Fibromyalgia

"Fibromyalgia … occurs most commonly in women twenty to fifty years old. The *National Institute of Arthritis and Musculoskeletal Diseases* estimates that five million people in the US suffer from the condition. Even though it's so widespread, the cause of fibromyalgia is still unclear."

Fibromyalgia Symptoms –
https://paindoctor.com/fibromyalgia-symptoms/

Fibromyalgia symptoms can include any or all of the following:

Widespread muscle soreness, muscle spasms, tenderness, headaches or migraines, rebound pain (a sensation of pain when pressure is removed), irritable bowel syndrome, nausea, constipation, diarrhea, painful bladder syndrome, pins and needles sensations, sensitivity to cold and to touch, forgetfulness, inability to concentrate, or "fibro fog," problems with balance and coordination, fatigue, depression, nervous energy, anxiety, emotional sensitivity, increased stress response, sleep disorders, joint stiffness, menstrual pain or changes.

Chronic Fatigue – CFS

People with chronic fatigue suffer with headaches, sleep disorders, memory and concentration problems, muscle pain, gastrointestinal problems, and pain in the joints. The severity of symptoms can vary widely from person to person.

Often, high levels of stress trigger this disorder, which usually starts with flu-like symptoms that do not improve over time. Continuing stressful events can worsen the symptoms, resulting in the person becoming bedridden. Chronic fatigue can persist for years, disrupting the individual's normal life and routine.

Adrenal Fatigue

Adrenal fatigue causes levels of a number of neuro-transmitters and hormones to lower. These changes can affect every part of the body.

An individual with adrenal fatigue will have most or all of these symptoms:
Difficulty getting up in the morning, high levels of fatigue, excessively stressed by stress, craving salty foods, higher energy levels in the evenings, dependence on caffeine and similar stimulants, a weak immune system, and for some, frequent urination, and low blood pressure.

Apple Cider Vinegar Helps These Conditions
Although apple cider vinegar is acidic, as previously mentioned it burns as alkaline ash in the body. In addition, it helps the digestive system and regulates blood sugar levels, two important areas that also need assistance for these three syndromes.

Emotional and physical anxiety causes lactic acid to accumulate in the body, resulting in exhaustion. The potassium in apple cider vinegar helps alleviate exhaustion.

Apple cider vinegar is effective in keeping the body's pH level slightly alkaline, contributing to eradicating headaches and joint pain, while acidosis is prevented by apple cider vinegar raising the pH, a major factor in pain management. It is also a natural blood thinner that helps move congested fluid in the body, which, of course, improves energy.

Apple cider vinegar kills viruses and bacteria. If consumed daily, joint aches and pains will gradually become less pronounced.

Malic Acid Boost
The malic acid in apple cider vinegar improves the flow of oxygen to muscle cells. The free radicals from oxidative stress are done away with by the trace nutrients in apple cider vinegar. There is as much as

twenty times more energy to go on after malic acid boosts muscles into better efficiency.

Apple cider vinegar contains calcium, sodium, magnesium, phosphorus, cilium, and potassium. These minerals are beneficial for people suffering from chronic fatigue syndrome, adrenal fatigue, and fibromyalgia, as they remove fatigue.

Rub apple cider vinegar on noticeably swollen areas to reduce swelling, and drink diluted apple cider vinegar for all the foregoing benefits, including alleviating swelling.

Apple Cider Vinegar & Food

Apple Cider Vinegar for Food Preservation
Not only cucumbers can be made into pickles! All sorts of fruits and vegetables can be preserved in apple cider vinegar. There are a variety of procedures from quick pickling, with picked produce that lasts for a month in the refrigerator, to full-on canning, with your beautiful fruits and veggies lined up on the shelf in your pantry.

Pickling preserves the food while adding a delightful *and healthy!* tang to the flavor. There are recipes that call for white vinegar, but use apple cider vinegar for its health advantage. The acetic acid in apple cider vinegar increases the acidity of the vegetables, which kills off any microorganisms and preserves the produce.

Apple Cider Vinegar for Food Poisoning
Apple cider vinegar is used as a treatment for food poisoning, easing the symptoms and supporting recovery. According to *The Natural Remedy Book for Women,* apple cider vinegar treatments annihilate the bacteria that make people sick. It is hydrating and also replaces vital nutrients and minerals lost due to vomiting and diarrhea.

Apple Cider Vinegar for Fungus
Fungal infections can affect your health in *so many* ways. Fungi cause various skin and nail disorders, such as athlete's foot, ringworm, urinary tract infections, pneumonia, and even meningitis. Let's take a detailed look at how to use apple cider vinegar in the management of mycosis.

Fungal infections are diseases caused by fungi, aka, molds. Or, more formally, mycosis. They can affect any part of the body, however, mycosis is most often found on skin and nails. They can also affect various internal organs and the brain, as in fungal meningitis.

Fungal Infections are Common
Fungal infections are quite common. For instance, athlete's foot, or *tinea pedis*, affects three to fifteen percent of the population. Candida, a yeast infec-

tion, affects about forty-six thousand people in the US.

Fungi grow when immune functions are compromised. Gut health is essential for the immune system to function properly. *Trillions* of supportive bacteria live in the digestive tract, capable of preventing disease-causing organisms, including fungi.

Apple Cider Vinegar Supports Good Bacteria
However, friendly bacteria need something to consume. If they are struggling to survive, they cannot grow, increasing the risk of fungal infection. Apple cider vinegar's acetic acid has antifungal power that eliminates microbes and fungi, while pectin supports good gut bacteria, which may, in turn, inhibit fungus growth.

Chlorogenic acid in apple cider vinegar inhibits the activity of oxidative stress of mycosis and inflammation-causing enzymes, like itching and redness. Along with pectin and acetic acid they put into full force antifungal power. Apply diluted or undiluted, according to your preference, apple cider vinegar to the nail and skin fungus directly.

Apple Cider Vinegar – Keep Your Gallbladder
The gallbladder is a small sac located just under the liver. It stores bile made by the liver to help digest fat. Bile

moves from the gallbladder to the small intestine through ductwork called the cystic duct or common bile duct.

The components in bile can crystallize and harden in the gallbladder, developing into gallstones. (Eighty percent of gallstones are made of cholesterol, and twenty percent are made of calcium salts and bilirubin, according to *Harvard Health Publications*.) Gallbladder attacks occur when gallstones block the movement of bile from the gallbladder.

However, millions of people have gallstones without any kind of pain whatsoever!

According to the *Florida Hospital*, only about three percent of people who suffer from painful gallstones actually develop inflammation, the leading cause of gallbladder removal.

Apple Cider Vinegar Stops Gallbladder Pain in its Tracks
Two to three tablespoons raw organic apple cider vinegar
Eight ounces apple cider or other juice
Drink within ten to fifteen minutes

Although it's common in the US to have gallbladders removed (cholecystectomy), please consider the following, and introduce apple cider vinegar into your daily routine, along with making some changes in dietary choices.

Gallbladder Surgery

Gallbladder surgery is a drastic step that alters digestion. Bile drips continuously into the digestive tract via the liver when there is no gallbladder gatekeeper. So, when bile is really needed to digest a fatty meal, there is almost none available. This leads to indigestion, poor absorption of healthy fats and fat-soluble vitamins, hormonal imbalance, and diarrhea … a domino effect of misery.

> *"Nearly one million gallbladders are removed every year in this country, and it is my estimate that only several thousand need to come out."*
> **Dr. Joseph Mercola**

Apple Cider Vinegar for Gout

Gout is on the rise in recent years due to the increase in obesity. Primarily middle-aged and older men are affected by it, but postmenopausal women are also experiencing gout. Debilitating pain in primarily the feet can prevent a person from going anywhere, or doing anything. Which only exacerbates the problem.

An excess of uric acid that enters the bloodstream and then crystallizes in the joints is the culprit that causes the joints to swell and become unbearably tender, the primary cause of gout.

But there is hope with apple cider vinegar, a wonderful natural remedy for gout that directly attacks the root cause. Let's look at how it works to ease the painful symptoms. Apple cider vinegar dissolves uric acid stones by binding with calcium, which is then excreted through urine. Malic acid dissolves the uric acid in the bloodstream, alleviating the worst of the symptoms, as apple cider vinegar's anti-inflammatory properties ease the swelling and pain of gout.

The abundant amount of potassium in apple cider vinegar helps remove waste from the body. The process of apple cider vinegar converting into alkaline ash helps it get rid of the toxic build-up, while at the same time it balances the pH of the internal environment. This process obliterates the symptoms of gout, while preventing the conditions that caused it.

Now, do your part and improve your diet, and *let's get physical!*

Apple Cider Vinegar & Gut Health

Digestive issues, gastrointestinal disease, irritable bowel syndrome (IBS), low stomach acid, and other stomach issues are becoming ever more common. This discomfort may include: abdominal pain, skin irritation, gas, constipation, and its pal, diarrhea, weight irregularities, weak immune system, and excessive bloating from the bacteria buildup.

Small intestinal bacterial overgrowth (SIBO), or other health concerns associated with an unbalanced gut microbiome leads to autoimmune problems, digestive problems, skin rashes or acne, sugar cravings, and poor sleep.

Due to its acidic nature and antimicrobial properties, apple cider vinegar increases stomach acid. This not only decreases bloating, but it helps break down and digest food, supporting healthy digestion and—*so important!*—nutrient absorption. Raw apple cider vinegar also contains pectin, a fiber that aids digestion, reduces stomach cramping and inflammation, and treats diarrhea resulting from irritable bowel syndrome.

Apple Cider Vinegar Slows Down Gastric Emptying
Apple cider vinegar has been shown to slow down gastric emptying, that is to say, slow the rate at which food leaves the stomach. This is extremely beneficial to those who suffer from IBS and other gut issues that cause irregular bowel movements. The whole digestive process is slowed down, calming diarrhea and reducing discomfort.

One-Hundred-Trillion Gut Bacteria
Our gut holds *one-hundred-trillion* good and bad bacteria, composed of between three-hundred to five-hundred

different kinds. The good bacteria have an important role not only in the gut, but are vital to our overall health. Keeping a well-balanced microbiota is essential. The Mother in apple cider vinegar has antimicrobial properties, able to destroy the spread of bad gut bacteria, while helping balance the microbiome. It's filled with friendly bacteria that improve the absorption of nutrients, improve immune health, and, *bonus!*, decrease sugar cravings.

Apple cider vinegar supports the gut bacteria with pepsin, a prebiotic that feeds the intestinal bacteria. Acetic acid changes the pH of the gut, and, in turn, makes pepsin more available. The pepsin feeds the bacteria in the gut, allowing the good bacteria to grow. The bacteria break down the pepsin into butyric acid, a short-chain fatty acid fuel for the gut. In addition to feeding your gut bacteria, it also heals the gut when it breaks down into a fatty acid that feeds the cells of the gut, which helps them to heal.

Apple Cider Vinegar's Acetic Acid Ramps Up Gut Motility

Not eating for a few hours allows the digestive system a chance to recover, and it's more able to burn fat. The acetic acid in apple cider vinegar digests food faster, ramps up the gut motility phase, and helps the thermogenic effect of white adipose tissue migrating to brown adipose tissue, which is then burned, resulting in weight loss.

Apple Cider Vinegar Fights Fungus & Bacteria & Aids in Detox & Regularity

Raw apple cider vinegar has antimicrobial effects against *E. coli, S aureus*, and *Candida albicans*. Raw apple cider vinegar helps reduce body fat and flushes out toxins, giving the gut a boost. Healthy gut bacteria are vital in maintaining bowel regularity. Apple cider vinegar boosts beneficial bacteria in the gut to prevent constipation.

Apple Cider Vinegar Boosts Nutrient Absorption

"An experiment with rats found that the absorption of calcium was higher when the rats were fed a diet containing apple cider vinegar for thirty-two days than when fed on a diet without vinegar."

> *Enhancing Effect of Dietary Vinegar on the*
> *Intestinal Absorption of Calcium in Rats –*
> *https://pubmed.ncbi.nlm.nih.gov/10380633/*

Apple Cider Vinegar & Traveling

Traveling is stressful, and stress causes inflammation, which is most often rooted in the gut. Taking apple cider vinegar before traveling feeds the gut bacteria so the stress of travel does not upset it, and also avoids bad bacteria manifesting, which is associated with weight gain. This might, in fact, have a significant role in the problem of weight gain while traveling.

A study from the *Journal of Crohn's and Colitis* found that high-altitude journeys and flights are associated with an increased risk of flares in inflammatory bowel disease patients. A lack of oxygen or the proverbial thin air, common at high altitudes or during flights, can trigger inflammation in the intestinal tract. Be sure to take apple cider vinegar before flying and after landing.

Apple Cider Vinegar for Hair

Apple cider vinegar contains enzymes, amino acids, and other nutrients that promote healthy hair. The pH level in apple cider vinegar helps restore the scalp to healthy pH levels, and its antibacterial properties remove buildup from other products. Among its many benefits are included improving the overall health of the scalp, which leads to shiny, healthy hair, and encourages hair growth.

Apple Cider Vinegar for Hair Loss

Apple cider vinegar helps with hair loss as the malic acid exfoliates the scalp, removing dead skin cells, augmenting blood circulation, and stimulating healthy, natural oils.

Mix a fifty-fifty solution of apple cider vinegar and water and apply evenly on damp or dry hair and then rinse off after five minutes. It penetrates deep into the strands and seals split ends.

Apple Cider Vinegar for Dandruff

Dandruff is a common problem. There are several causes for a flaky and itchy scalp. It's caused by a fungus called Malassezia, normally present on the scalp, but various irritants such as pollution, improper hygiene, or hormonal changes make the fungus produce a bi-product called oleic acid.

The acid triggers excess skin cells shedding, on which the fungus feeds. Apple cider vinegar can help alleviate dandruff symptoms naturally, as the enzymes and probiotics it contains are capable of eradicating both bacterial and fungal infections. Its anti-inflammatory properties soothe the swelling and irritation of the dandruff infection.

Apple cider vinegar's enzymes open clogged pores, making the scalp healthy, adding shine and volume to hair. It helps restore the scalp's healthy moisture level, while the acidic acid maintains pH balance, removing build-up without stripping the hair of its natural oils. By restoring the natural pH of the scalp, fungus, bacteria, and yeast will not consider it a suitable home.

Treatment

Mix one-quarter cup of apple cider vinegar with one-quarter cup of water and work it into the scalp. Wrap your hair in a towel, allowing the mixture to remain on the scalp for fifteen minutes, then wash the hair as usual.

Apple Cider Vinegar for Headaches

Headaches have numerous causes, ranging from allergies and digestive issues to stress and high blood pressure. There are tension headaches, cluster headaches, sinus headaches, hormonal headaches, and tension headaches, to name a few.

Apple cider vinegar works on the underlying cause or causes of headaches. It contains iron, potassium, and calcium. These minerals and acids help reduce headaches. The potassium in apple cider vinegar also helps treat migraine pain.

Apple cider vinegar aids digestion, which helps prevent headaches caused by digestive issues. It reduces blood sugar levels in subjects with diabetes. This benefit regulates blood sugar spikes, which sometimes cause headaches.

Inhaling vaporized apple cider vinegar can help clear out the sinuses and relieve a sinus headache. Dehydration is another common cause of headaches. Adding a tablespoon of apple cider vinegar to a glass of water stimulates hydration.

Apple Cider Vinegar for Heartburn

Two of the primary causes of heartburn and acid reflux are an improper balance in the pH of the stomach, as well as a lack of probiotics and enzymes. Apple cider vinegar is loaded with these nutrients and can ease the burning sensation in the chest that is caused by heartburn and acid reflux. Drink one or two tablespoons of apple cider vinegar in a glass of water before eating to prevent the onset of heartburn and indigestion.

How does apple cider vinegar's acid calm heartburn and acid reflux? Not because there is too much acid in the stomach, but because there is *too little*. Apple cider vinegar strengthens the stomach acid and arrests acid reflux and heartburn from junk food. *But don't eat junk food!*

Apple Cider Vinegar for Heat Exhaustion

Apple cider vinegar is rich in essential minerals as well as vitamins. It helps the body retrieve lost electrolytes. A glass of cool water with one to three teaspoons of apple cider vinegar added will overcome heat exhaustion and its attendant feelings of weakness and fatigue.

Apple Cider Vinegar for Hiccups

Apple cider vinegar stimulates the transient receptor potential (TRP) channels in the mouth. Activating these receptors overwhelms the muscle contractions that lead to hiccups. This mechanism explains why apple cider vinegar can stop hiccups immediately. Just a sip or two will halt hiccups.

Apple Cider Vinegar for Hot Flashes

A hot flash begins as a sudden sensation of intense heat involving the face and upper chest, rapidly involving the entire body. The sensation may be accompanied by profuse sweating, chills, palpitations, and anxiety. Frequency varies from occasional attacks during a week to a couple of times an hour. They often present as night sweats, accompanied by sleep disturbances. Severe hot flashes can interfere with the activities of daily living, having a negative impact on quality of life.

Although hot flashes cannot be prevented, they can be curbed with apple cider vinegar, which contains antioxidants, enzymes, and healthy bacteria, that assist in flushing out toxins. Extensive clinical research has shown how apple cider vinegar works to eliminate toxins from the body, the same toxins the body is trying to eliminate through sweating during hot flashes. Apple cider vinegar reduces the frequency and severity of hot flashes and alleviates sweating and discomfort.

Since apple cider vinegar aids in alkalinizing the body, it assists with the natural alleviation of hot flashes and night sweats. It is rich in magnesium, essential for bone mass, and for enhancing the healthy functioning of nerves. It also contributes to stabilizing mood swings, stress, and depression.

The detoxifying nature of the anti-inflammatory properties of apple cider vinegar is also enhanced by daily physical exercise. The standard dosage of one teaspoon to two tablespoons, one to three times per day, starting low and increasing until you find your "comfort spot" is recommended.

Apple Cider Vinegar for Hypertension & Heart Health

Taking apple cider vinegar for high blood pressure may be a very good natural solution to manage the entirely too common health condition of hypertension.

"A recent study estimated that globally, thirty-two percent of women and thirty-four percent of men between the ages of thirty and seventy-nine have the condition—that's over a billion people."
https://healthmatch.io/high-blood-pressure/how-many-people-have-high-blood-pressure

And in the US, about one in three adults has high blood pressure, which includes almost half of the people over sixty-five years of age.

The main component of apple cider vinegar, acetic acid, is beneficial for reducing high blood pressure by balancing the body's pH. Breaking down phlegm deposits and fat in the body can lead to lower pressure against the arterial walls and better overall circulation.

A study published in the *British Journal of Nutrition* showed that the acetic acid in apple cider vinegar could effectively control high blood pressure by reducing cholesterol in rats. The group taking acetic acid in their diet had significantly lower triglyceride and cholesterol levels.

Metabolic Syndrome

Having high triglycerides in the blood is linked to atherosclerosis, a thickening of the artery wall due to plaque buildup. High triglycerides may also be a sign of metabolic syndrome—a combination of high triglycerides, high blood pressure, high blood sugar, low HDL (high-density lipoprotein) cholesterol, and a large waist circumference of too much fat.

High LDL cholesterol is associated with high blood pressure. When there is too much LDL cholesterol in the blood, the arteries become narrow and harden with cholesterol, and the heart must work extra hard to pump blood through these narrow, inflexible halls.

Various studies have shown that apple cider vinegar is capable of significantly reducing both triglycerides and blood pressure. A little reminder, raw apple cider vinegar is *the only vinegar that is alkaline-forming in the body*. All other kinds of vinegars are acid-forming.

Improving Blood Circulation

Apple cider vinegar eliminates toxins and pollutants from the blood and promotes healthy blood circulation. It helps stabilize blood pressure whether it is too high or too low.

A large observational study found that people who ate oil and apple cider vinegar dressing on salads five to six times a week had lower rates of heart disease than people who didn't. It's just that simple.

The potassium in apple cider vinegar is beneficial to both the heart and normalizing blood pressure by helping make the blood thinner, resulting in a reduction of high blood pressure.

In a study performed on laboratory animals, apple cider vinegar improved the ability of heart cells to repair themselves (*impressive!*) after being damaged by free radicals.

Apple Cider Vinegar for Infections, Cuts, & Wounds

With its powerful antibacterial, antimicrobial, and antifungal properties, apple cider vinegar can be used to clean wounds and kill bacteria. Its acetic acid kills the bacteria and heals the infection while boosting the immune system to fight against infection.

To use apple cider vinegar on a wound or cut, apply a cloth soaked in a one-to-one apple cider vinegar solution on the wound. Repeat this process several times a day until the wound heals. To aid in healing, drink the standard suggested treatment: a glass of water with one-to-two tablespoons of apple cider vinegar in it, one to three times per day.

Apple Cider Vinegar for Insomnia

Aside from drinking apple cider vinegar first thing in the morning, it is also a good idea to have some before going to bed. It provides the following benefits:

Helps Manage Blood Glucose

Apple cider vinegar slows down the movement and emptying of our intestines. This helps prevent glucose spikes while sleeping.

Insulin resistance or the inability to produce insulin is what characterizes type 2 diabetes. Apple cider vinegar helps manage blood glucose for diabetics … and for everyone.

It has been shown that apple cider vinegar improves sensitivity to insulin even with a high-carb meal. Apple cider vinegar at night reduces fasting blood sugar the next morning.

Antimicrobial Properties
Apple cider vinegar has antimicrobial properties that cut down the bacteria called *Helicobacter pylori,* which causes bad breath in the morning.

Better Breathing
Apple cider vinegar will also help support a better respiratory system. It allows more oxygen to be absorbed for healthier breathing while sleeping, and it stimulates hormone secretion, optimizing the metabolic system.

Refreshing Sleep
A good night's sleep pays off when waking up refreshed and in a great frame of mind!

Apple Cider Vinegar and Kidney Stones
Kidney stones are hard deposits composed of salts, minerals, and other substances that develop when urine contains too much calcium and/or uric acid. Kidney stones cause the blood plasma to thicken.

Ancient Cure for Our Modern Ailment
Apple cider vinegar has been used to treat kidney stones for thousands of years. In addition to helping

dissolve kidney stones, or, even better, prevent them from forming in the first place, apple cider vinegar is a helpful healing solution. The acetic acid, malic acid, and pectin in apple cider vinegar treat and prevent kidney stones.

The severe pain associated with kidney stones and the accompanying bladder spasms may be reduced by apple cider vinegar, which neutralizes excess acid in the urine. Apple cider vinegar kills disease-producing bacteria in the kidneys and bladder, and the debris is flushed out naturally.

Apple cider vinegar is a natural diuretic, increasing the amount of urine produced, helping to flush out small stones, and preventing them from getting stuck in the kidney tubes or ureter. Further, blood pressure is regulated when there is less fluid retention.

How Apple Cider Vinegar Dissolves Kidney Stones

The crystals that cause kidney stones are softened by the citric acid in apple cider vinegar, and they easily pass from the body. One of the causes of kidney stones is dehydration. This results in less urine. A daily dose of apple cider vinegar encourages the body to produce more urine that flushes the stone-making minerals.

And, drink enough water!

One study showed that drinking two tablespoons of apple cider vinegar three times a day resulted in forty percent fewer stones. But even more impressive, kidney stones were prevented from forming in the first place. Why? Because of lowered levels of phosphorus, oxalate, and calcium.

In an experiment that involved twenty men suffering with kidney stones, half of them drank two tablespoons of apple cider vinegar in water, three times a day for three months. The other half received a placebo of the same dose for three months. This study had significant positive results, with the men who drank apple cider vinegar producing *twenty-six percent* more urine than those who took the placebo and lowering their calcium by ten percent.

Healthy Digestion with the Aid of Apple Cider Vinegar
Apple cider vinegar is known to have several digestive benefits, including regulating citric acid. It also helps reduce gas, constipation, and bloating. Most people who suffer with kidney stones tend to experience all these digestive problems.

Though apple cider vinegar isn't particularly high in calcium, the acetic acid that it contains helps the body's ability to absorb more minerals, including calcium.

Reduce Cystitis & Prostatitis with Apple Cider Vinegar
Taking apple cider vinegar on a daily basis helps reduce the pain and improve bladder control and blood flow associated with cystitis and prostatitis. It also helps bring the body's pH levels into balance, contributing to both pain reduction and good health.

Apple cider vinegar aids digestion by stimulating the production of hydrochloric acid (HCL) in the stomach. This helps break down food while killing bacteria and viruses. Acetic acid also kills micro-organisms that cause yeast infections, bloating, indigestion, and intestinal gas.

NOTE:
Avoid medications that may promote stone growth, such as calcium channel blockers used to treat high blood pressure when treating urinary tract stones with acetic acid.

Apple Cider Vinegar for Leg Cramps
Though the exact cause of restless leg is unknown, some believe that low potassium levels are to blame. Because apple cider vinegar has high amounts of potassium, it helps to reduce leg cramps.

Try a glass of water with a couple of tablespoons of apple cider vinegar to successfully alleviate leg cramps.

Apple Cider Vinegar for Lice

Anyone can be "lousy," but, in particular, six to twelve million children between the ages of three to eleven suffer from lice infestation in the US annually.

Apple cider vinegar is an outstanding natural treatment to eradicate lice. After washing the hair with a medicated shampoo specifically for eliminating lice, pour apple cider vinegar on the scalp and cover with a towel or shower cap and leave it on for ten minutes. Then comb the hair with a lice comb and rinse. This process kills lice by dissolving the glue they secrete, and the acid of apple cider vinegar kills the larvae.

The antiseptic and anti-inflammatory properties of apple cider vinegar heal the sores on the scalp.

Apple Cider Vinegar for Liver Health

The liver is a blood purifier, it helps remove toxins and waste substances from the blood, and it extracts nutrients. When the liver is not functioning properly, blood circulation is sluggish. Apple cider vinegar helps improve blood circulation and repairs damaged cells.

Fatty liver disease is a metabolic disorder caused by a combination of unhealthy lifestyle and genetic factors. A study with laboratory rats revealed that apple send her vinegar improves the fat-burning process in the liver. The liver becomes more sensitive to insulin, which increases the rate of burning fat inside liver cells.

Apple cider vinegar can help a damaged or diseased liver process sugars, fats, and cholesterol. The results of a study conducted on fifteen women with elevated cholesterol showed that the group who consumed daily apple cider vinegar had lower levels of harmful lipids in their blood compared to the control group.

Apple Cider Vinegar Improves Insulin Sensitivity

Type 2 diabetes is a metabolic disorder resulting from cells that are no longer sensitive to insulin. Many patients with diabetes may suffer from fatty liver disease because the high glucose level in the blood damages liver cells, causing them to accumulate excess fat. Apple cider vinegar can help.

There are two types of fatty liver disease: alcoholic fatty liver disease, caused by an excess of alcohol, and nonalcoholic fatty liver disease (NAFLD) or Nonalcoholic SteatoHepatitis (NASH), caused by a diet too rich in sugars. Over eighty million people in the US have fatty liver disease.

Daily apple cider vinegar helps with weight loss, reduces cholesterol levels, lowers blood sugar levels, and improves insulin sensitivity, all of which contribute to reducing the risk of getting type 2 diabetes. Apple cider vinegar improves digestion and is capable of balancing acidity in the body. It also facilitates metabolism, the elimination of toxins, and helps prevent damage caused by free radicals.

Apple Cider Vinegar Lowers Triglycerides & Increases HDL
Patients with elevated triglyceride levels are more likely to have nonalcoholic fatty liver disease. The results of a study showed that drinking two tablespoons of apple cider vinegar in eight ounces of water before each meal for sixteen weeks lowered triglyceride levels by ten percent, and increased HDL levels by seven percent.

As previously mentioned, HDL, the good cholesterol, helps lower triglycerides and LDL, the bad cholesterol that causes plaque to form inside arteries and increases the risk of high blood pressure, stroke, and heart attack.

In a laboratory study, mice were fed a high-fat diet. The group that was given apple cider vinegar had a higher level of HDL than the group that consumed only high-fat foods, demonstrating, at least in this study, that apple cider vinegar increased good cholesterol more effectively than grape seed extract.

Apple Cider Vinegar Reduces Inflammation
in the Digestive Tract
Inflammation in the digestive tract can cause fatty liver disease. The inflammation is caused by a lack of good gut microbiome, often due to excessive consumption of

sugar and fried foods. Apple cider vinegar can improve the digestion process and reduce the amount of sugar in the blood. It also helps reduce fat absorption from food. By improving the digestion process, the body is able to absorb more beneficial nutrients from food.

The inability to break down excessive amounts of fat accumulated in the liver is a result of poor diet and physical inactivity. Therefore, *and you've heard this before*, apple cider vinegar will work best when combined with exercise and a healthy diet.

Apple Cider Vinegar & the Lymph System

The lymph nodes are designed to protect the body from disease, as the lymphatic system clears out the excess interstitial fluid. This is extremely important to the overall health of the body. In order to do this, it's important to keep movement in the circulatory system. Stagnation is the way to dysfunction, disorders, and disease. Movement in the circulatory system means movement of the body. The lymph system does not have a heart moving lymph around. You must do it yourself!

Chronic stress, acute or chronic infections, toxin accumulation, dehydration, nutrient deficiencies, and a sedentary lifestyle all contribute to a sluggish, unhealthy lymphatic system. Pain and swelling are the result when bacterial infections build up in the lymph nodes. These bacteria must get flushed out of the body!

Apple cider vinegar helps break up mucus and cleanse the lymph nodes. Drinking one to three teaspoons of apple cider vinegar in a glass of warm water two or three times a day will reduce swelling in the lymph nodes. Soaking in a bath with a cup of apple cider vinegar added will also help to fight infection, clear lymphatic congestion, and reduce the swelling and pain in the lymph nodes.

Apple Cider Vinegar for Malaria

Malaria is an infectious disease in red blood cells caused by a protozoan of the genus *Plasmodium*. It is characterized by cycles of fever, chills, and sweating. The disease is transmitted to humans by the bite of an infected female anopheles mosquito.

Apple cider vinegar is a known antipyretic (prevent or allay fever) that will help you combat fever. A cloth dipped in apple cider vinegar and water and placed on the forehead will reduce fever, as well as the standard one or two tablespoons in a glass of water, which will contribute to the healing process while reducing nausea and vomiting.

Apple Cider Vinegar and Making Baby

Apple cider vinegar is great for improving your health in several areas. It restores the body's normal pH balance, and its anti-inflammatory attribute benefits fertility. Drinking apple cider vinegar in water improves the gut environment, which directly affects and improves the entire internal environment.

Avoid products that contain harmful toxins and chemicals such as BPA, parabens, propylene glycol, and sodium lauryl sulfate, which can be detrimental to fertility. Use beauty and grooming products with natural ingredients, including apple cider vinegar.

Apple cider vinegar treats yeast infections, which can cause a variety of issues that upset fertility. It can help treat polycystic ovary syndrome. Women with PCOS have higher testosterone levels, but apple cider vinegar lowers those levels.

A woman's vaginal pH needs to be at a level of four to five. When the pH is higher or lower, it can disrupt fertility. Apple cider vinegar contributes to controlling this pH level.

And apple cider vinegar helps strengthen and nourish a man's sperm and makes for better motility.

Apple Cider Vinegar for Morning Sickness

Apple cider vinegar is made through fermentation and is very helpful for treating morning sickness. Many women have reported eliminating morning sickness simply by adding apple cider vinegar to their drinking water.

Apple Cider Vinegar for Nerve Pain

Apple cider vinegar has been shown to help relieve nerve pain, whether caused by diabetic neuropathy, back injury, sciatica, multiple sclerosis, multiple myeloma, cancer, diabetes, autoimmune illness, physical trauma, chemicals, poisons, excessive alcohol consumption, or even cancer treatment itself. Diabetic rats were given apple cider vinegar and subsequently had less diabetic neuropathy.

Low potassium levels cause weak nerve signals, resulting in tingling or numbness. Increase potassium with apple cider vinegar.

Apple cider vinegar's nutrient-rich makeup of magnesium, calcium, phosphorous, potassium, malic acid, and acetic acid assists in its powerful anti-inflammatory, antibacterial, and antifungal effects to treat neuropathic pain. A toxin called guanidine, a by-product of metabolism, causes nerve pain. Apple cider vinegar binds with it and reduces nerve pain.

One possible treatment for neuropathic pain relief is soaking your feet for thirty minutes in a one-to-two apple cider vinegar to water ratio.

Apple Cider Vinegar for Obesity

Researchers have looked into the specific compounds in apple cider vinegar that may be responsible for improving oxidative stress and significantly reducing the risk of obesity. Numerous studies have shown that it helps lower the risk of obesity by reducing oxidative stress and preventing fat accumulation.

Tunisian Obesity Researchers

A group of researchers in Tunisia wanted to see if taking apple cider vinegar daily would affect cardiovascular risk factors associated with obesity in obese rats fed a high-fat diet. The rats had increased levels of triglycerides and low-density lipoprotein (LDL).

The rats developed oxidative stress—which occurs when there is an imbalance between free radical formation and the capability of cells to clear them—after six weeks of being fed the high-fat diet. Free radicals are reactive molecules that damage healthy cells and their components. Obesity is characterized by chronic low-grade inflammation with permanently increased oxidative stress levels.

The researchers orally administered apple cider vinegar to the treatment rats. At the end of the experiment, the rats that received apple cider vinegar had lower total cholesterol, triglyceride, and LDL levels than the controls. Apple cider vinegar also improved oxidative stress and normalized various metabolic changes brought on by the high-fat diet.

Japanese Obesity Researchers

Researchers from Japan looked into the effects of acetic acid on the processes that convert food into body fat. They began by feeding mice fatty foods to induce obesity. The mice were then divided into a control group and two treatment groups.

The control group of mice was daily given water for six weeks, while the treatment groups received either a 0.3 percent or a 1.5 percent dose of acetic acid. After the treatment period, the researchers collected blood and liver samples and measured the amount of body fat and liver fat in the samples. They also cultivated human HepG2 liver cells and added acetic acid to the culture.

The control mice had clear symptoms of obesity, but the mice treated with acetic acid did not become obese. The researchers reported that acetic acid stopped body fat from accumulating and also seemed to have prevented the formation of excess fat in the liver.

Apple Cider Vinegar for Poison-Oak/Poison-Ivy/ Poison Sumac

Poison oak, poison ivy, and poison sumac are found in most parts of the United States. A painful rash develops when a person comes in contact with any one of these plants. The culprit is urushiol—an oil produced by leaves and stems of poison ivy, oak, or sumac plants. The rash spreads rapidly in the initial days. The severity of the rash depends on the exposure to the urushiol.

Vinegar Compress

An apple cider vinegar compress dries out the blisters and reduces itching. Use a somewhat strong solution of one-half cup of apple cider vinegar to one-and-one-half cup of water. Soak a cloth in the mixture and apply to the affected area, leaving it on for two to five minutes. Repeat as necessary until the rash is healed.

Apple Cider Vinegar for Pneumonia

Apple cider vinegar is an effective home remedy for pneumonia with its powerful antibacterial, antiviral, and antifungal properties that triumph over bacterial, viral, or fungal pneumonia. Its anti-inflammatory property helps it combat the respiratory inflammation in the lungs.

Take the recommended oral dosage of one to three tablespoons in a glass of warm water two or three times a day until symptoms resolve.

Apple Cider Vinegar for Stress Reduction

Stress can cause many diseases, like high blood pressure, depression, diabetes, obesity, and even cancer. Apple cider vinegar has been found to be effective in reducing blood pressure and heart rate. Apple cider vinegar can lower stress hormone levels by eighty percent, according to the *Chinese Medicine Institute*.

But don't take too much too fast when you're starting. There are reports from individual people that apple cider vinegar causes them the opposite of reduced stress and made them feel anxious. Decreasing the amount of apple cider vinegar generally resolves this reaction.

Apple Cider Vinegar for Skin

Apple cider vinegar can help clear up skin conditions and blemishes.

Acne & Age Spots

Kill acne and fade age spots by using apple cider vinegar as a skin toner. The antibacterial properties of apple cider vinegar help keep acne under control. It is even superior to other products which may dry out the skin or cause other adverse effects.

The lactic and malic acids in apple cider vinegar help to soften and exfoliate the skin. A cloth saturated in apple cider vinegar after washing the face will reveal a brighter, less blemished complexion. It's also helpful for removing pore-clogging debris that can lead to acne.

Apple Cider Vinegar for Eczema

Eczema is a term for a variety of conditions that can cause skin to become inflamed, red, or itchy. More than thirty-one million Americans suffer from some type of eczema. Common symptoms of eczema include itchy, dry, sensitive skin, with areas of swelling.

Healthy skin is protected by an acidic barrier. Researchers believe that this acidic barrier doesn't work properly for people with eczema. This is because people with eczema have elevated pH levels in their skin. Healthy skin has a pH level under five. People with eczema have a pH level over five.

If the acidic skin barrier isn't working properly, moisture escapes from the skin, and irritants enter the body. Skin acidity can also be influenced by the skin's own microbiota, protection against bacteria. There are higher levels of staph bacteria on the skin of people who have eczema.

The reason apple cider vinegar works for eczema is that it is a mild acid, and it helps adjust the skin's pH to a healthy level. Apple cider vinegar has been used as an alternative treatment for eczema for decades. The acid in apple cider vinegar reduces both bacteria and yeast in the skin.

Members of the *National Eczema Association* have reported that apple cider vinegar baths are soothing to the skin and boost its moisture levels.

Apple Cider Vinegar for Psoriasis

Psoriasis is a chronic condition that causes skin cells to grow rapidly, with resulting dry, scaly patches of raised, red skin. The skin may burn, flake, itch, or sting. It may be just a small patch or patches on the surface of the skin, but it can also grow over much of the body.

Apple cider vinegar is a wonderful treatment for psoriasis, both internally and externally. *The National Psoriasis Foundation* (NPF) endorses apple cider vinegar as a treatment to help stop itching.

Improves Wrinkles

The use of malic acid for skin care products is not uncommon. Due to its antioxidant and exfoliation benefits, it's commonly used for a range of skin concerns, including fine lines and wrinkles, hyperpigmentation, acne, large pores, milia, warts, and calluses.

Malic acid is an extremely effective skin refiner, as it stimulates the shedding of the outer layer of skin cells, which process has anti-aging effects.

Apple Cider Vinegar for Diaper Rash
Infantile seborrheic dermatitis is a condition that results in inflammatory scaling skin. It causes skin rashes in the diaper area. Apple cider vinegar helps remove the inflammation and the scales.

Add a teaspoon of apple cider vinegar to half-a-cup of water and gently clean the diaper area. Apply a few times a day for results in a few days of continuous usage.

Apple Cider Vinegar for Sunburn
Soaking in the bath with a cup or two of apple cider vinegar added to the water can soothe the pain of a sunburn, and help heal it. Apple cider vinegar's anti-inflammatory properties work to reduce the inflammation of the sunburn.

Apple Cider Vinegar for Soreness After a Workout
Muscle pain and fatigue at the gym can often be symptoms of underlying conditions that begin to manifest during times of extended stress on muscles. It's suggested to drink apple cider vinegar before working out as its vitamins, and minerals will balance pH levels, improve stamina, decrease muscle fatigue, and minimize muscle pain. Balanced pH monitors carbon diox-

ide and contributes to oxygenating the body when under stress.

The buildup of lactic acid in the body can cause fatigue. The amino acids in apple cider vinegar serve as an antidote. Additionally, the enzymes and potassium in apple cider vinegar help to relieve tiredness.

Exercise-induced muscle cramps aren't always a sign of muscle exhaustion. They also indicate calcium, magnesium, or potassium deficiencies caused by electrolyte imbalances. Because apple cider vinegar has high amounts of potassium, it helps to reduce leg cramps.

The National Center for Alternative and Complementary Medicine has stated that lactose intolerance, intestinal viruses, parasites, and alcohol all potentially contribute to exercise-induced muscle fatigue. Taking apple cider vinegar before going to the gym helps prevent muscle cramps by replenishing electrolytes.

Malic Acid
Apple cider vinegar's malic acid produces energy through the breakdown of fat calories. It also increases energy by dissolving toxins that cause fatigue and weakness. Further, research on its role in weight loss shows that it speeds up metabolism.

A Swedish pharmacist by the name of Carl Wilhelm Scheele discovered malic acid in apples in 1785. The name malic comes from the Latin name of apple, which is *malum*.

Malic acid and acetic acid play an important role in the Krebs cycle, an energy-producing sequence of reactions. The Krebs cycle metabolizes carbohydrates, proteins, and fatty acids, producing adenosine triphosphate, ATP.

Malic Acid Promotes Better Exercise Performance
Malic acid is taken as a supplement to boost athletic performance and discourage post-exercise muscle fatigue. Sometimes it's taken in conjunction with creatine, a popular supplement to increase lean muscle mass.

A study published in *Acta Physiologica Hungarica* looked at the effects of a creatine malate supplement in long-distance runners, as well as sprinters. After six weeks of supplementation along with their physical training, a significant increase in growth hormone was observed in the sprinter group. Notably, both sprinters and long-distance runners experienced improved physical performance. There was a significant increase in the distance the long-distance runners were able to run.

Apple Cider Vinegar for Strong Teeth & Healthy Mouth
The antibacterial properties of apple cider vinegar kill the bacteria in the mouth and throat that cause cavities,

gum disease, and bad breath, and the potassium in apple cider vinegar strengthens teeth.

Apple cider vinegar is known for its ability to whiten teeth. Dip your toothbrush in apple cider vinegar and brush gently for a minute, then rinse thoroughly. Only do this a couple of times a week at the most so that the acid does not harm the enamel.

Malic Acid Improves Oral Health
Research had demonstrated that malic acid can improve symptoms of dry mouth by stimulating saliva production. Healthy saliva production also helps prevent the overgrowth of oral bacteria.

Apple Cider Vinegar for Ulcers
The most common sites for ulcers are the stomach and mouth. The lacerations and scars of ulcers cause extreme pain. The pain of canker sores causes limited movement of the mouth, making it difficult to talk and eat. Mouth ulcers will heal naturally, but they can take a long time.

Apple cider vinegar reduces the time of healing, while being safe and effective. It helps relieve the pain of stomach ulcers by correcting the stomach's pH balance. It's especially effective in treating peptic ulcers, killing the *H. pylori* bacteria that causes ulcers, and the vitamins, minerals, and probiotics ease the other painful effects of peptic ulcers.

As always, be sure to dilute the apple cider vinegar. Undiluted, it can be extremely painful on open canker sores, as well as damage the esophagus.

Apple Cider Vinegar for Varicose Veins

Varicose veins and vein disease occur because the tiny valves, flaps of tissue inside the vein, stop functioning properly. Valves prevent blood from flowing backward in the pause between heartbeats, with the result that blood pools in the veins which then becomes distended, especially in the lower legs. While many people have no symptoms, others experience leg pain, swelling, burning, and itching. When severe, the skin over a vein may develop ulcers, especially with people who have diabetes.

Apple cider vinegar improves blood flow and circulation and cleanses the body of toxins. The recommendation is to apply undiluted apple cider vinegar to the skin over the varicose veins and gently massage into the skin twice a day. Also recommended is drinking two teaspoons of apple cider vinegar in a glass of water, twice a day. Apple cider vinegar has antioxidant properties that combat free radicals, which damage molecules that affect the body's cells.

One study examined eighty patients with varicose veins. The half of the participants who applied fabric wraps soaked with apple cider vinegar to their legs for thirty minutes, morning and night while their legs were kept elevated, resulted in relief from pain, itching, cramping, and swelling of the legs by the end of the study.

Apple Cider Vinegar for Vertigo
A sensation of dizzying, whirling motion in the surroundings, which may be caused by disorders of the inner ear. Apple cider vinegar significantly improves symptoms of vertigo after dosing with one tablespoon and a glass of warm water on a daily basis. It also increases blood circulation, relieves headaches, and boosts the immune system, while maintaining stable blood glucose levels following a meal ... all of which can improve vertigo.

Apple Cider Vinegar for Warts, Moles, Boils, Foot Corns & Ringworm
Warts, which are contagious, occur when the human papillomavirus (HPV) penetrates the uppermost protective layer of skin. There are more than one-hundred-fifty types of this common virus. Most forms of HPV are spread by casual skin contact or through shared objects, such as towels and washcloths.

A nevus, or mole, is a dark brown spot, caused by clusters of pigment-forming cells (melanocytes). Some moles are present at birth, while others develop over the course of a lifetime. Most moles are harmless.

A boil is a very sore, red, swollen bump surrounded by red, irritated skin. Usually, one or more heads, called pustules, will form in the center, filled with a pus-like fluid. Sometimes boils heal without forming a whitehead. A boil that develops multiple heads is called a carbuncle. Though it's a temptation to squeeze it, this is strongly advised against, as it can cause the infection to go into the body and potentially become serious.

Foot corns are areas of skin that have become thicker than the surrounding skin due to friction. They may be extremely painful and affect the deeper layers of skin. Corns are circular or cone-shaped.

Ringworm is a contagious fungal infection caused by mold-like parasites that live in cells in the outer layer of skin. It spreads by direct skin-to-skin contact with an infected person or animal.

The antibacterial properties of apple cider vinegar help get rid of all of these afflictions and keep them from spreading. Treat warts, moles, boils, foot corns, and ringworm by soaking a cloth in apple cider vinegar and placing it on the affected area, securing it with a band-aid. Leave it on overnight and repeat until the condition resolves.

Apple Cider Vinegar for Weight Loss

If food is not metabolized efficiently, nutrients are not accessible, which results in excess weight gain. Apple cider vinegar helps the digestion process while detoxifying the body. The result is a highly efficient metabolism that burns fat so that the body uses it rather than stores it. Apple cider vinegar also reduces appetite, minimizing the intake of food.

A study that investigated the effects of apple cider vinegar's acetic acid on reducing body fat mass in obese Japanese for twelve weeks, discovered that the intake of acetic acid was beneficial in lowering not only body weight, but also, the body mass index (BMI), waist circumference (WC), and visceral fat, along with levels of serum triglycerides in the participants involved in the study. *Impressive!*

In yet another study, obese people were divided into two groups. One group took apple cider vinegar while eating and the other drank water. At the end of the study, those who took the apple cider vinegar lost up to two pounds.

Apple Cider Vinegar Reduces Hunger

Satiety has been measured in response to white bread and various doses of vinegar. There was a progressive relationship between the satiety score and the amount of vinegar ingested in another study. Further, it was discovered that daily doses of apple cider vinegar resulted in an intake of between 200-275 fewer calories throughout the day.

Scientists hypothesize that apple cider vinegar interferes with the digestion of starches, inhibiting salivary amylase, which specifically interferes with carbohydrate absorption. There's also the fact that apple cider vinegar slows gastric emptying.

Metabolic syndrome is a serious consequence of obesity, characterized by increased cardiovascular risk factors such as hypertension, dyslipidemia, and glucose intolerance. This study tested whether a daily dosage of apple cider vinegar would affect cardiovascular risk factors associated with obesity in high-fat diet-induced hyperlipidemic Wistar rats.

Apple Cider Vinegar Suppresses Obesity-Induced Oxidative Stress

The obese rats developed increased serum total cholesterol, triglyceride, low-density lipoprotein-cholesterol (LDL-C), very-low-density lipoprotein (VLDL), and atherogenic index after six and nine weeks of being fed a high-fat diet.

Apple cider vinegar ameliorated all of these parameters significantly, showing that it can be beneficial for the suppression of obesity-induced oxidative stress in high-fat diet rats by modulating the antioxidant defense system, reducing the risk of obesity-associated diseases.

An important overall insight is that apple cider vinegar not only displaces carbohydrate calories but it also positively affects the insulin response.

Apple Cider Vinegar's Acidic Acid & Fasting

Insulin will spike whenever *anything* is eaten, no matter how little, and the body will never burn fat while eating. When insulin levels calm down after eating, fatty acids are activated and burned, which is why fasting is effective.

A study by the *Journal of Agriculture and Food Chemistry* showed that apple cider vinegar's acetic acid activated PPAR Alpha (peroxisome proliferator-activated receptor alpha), which is the master switch that allows the body to utilize and burn fats better.

It drives up AMPK (adenosine monophosphate-activated protein kinase), an enzyme that, when activated, tells the body to tap into stored body fat tissues, and to activate autophagy (clearing out damaged cells), thus making the fast restorative, and moving the body into a fasting state *faster*.

Interestingly, acidic acid also *turns down* AMPK in the brain, with the result of feeling less hungry. So, while the body is burning fat, you're feeling less hungry.

Simply put, apple cider vinegar, when used in conjunction with fasting, helps you achieve your health and weight loss goals faster, while improving insulin sensitivity, decreasing cravings, and decreasing inflammation.

Chapter High Points:

1. Tumor cells die on exposure to acetic acid.

2. Apple cider vinegar's antioxidants fight cell-damaging free radicals.

3. An apple cider vinegar poultice or soak can alleviate and even eradicate pain for ailments from itching, to rashes, to cuts, to neuropathic pain, to arthritis, and beyond.

4. Apple cider vinegar's immune-boosting probiotics of yeast and good bacteria in the Mother eliminate infections.

5. Apple cider vinegar helps reduce LDL cholesterol and boosts HDL cholesterol.

6. Apple cider vinegar lowers glucose.

7. Apple cider vinegar's probiotics and enzymes reduce heartburn and acid reflux.

8. Apple cider vinegar's acetic acid body absorbs more minerals.

9. Apple cider vinegar helps cleanse the lymph system.

10. The high level of potassium in apple cider vinegar helps balance electrolytes.

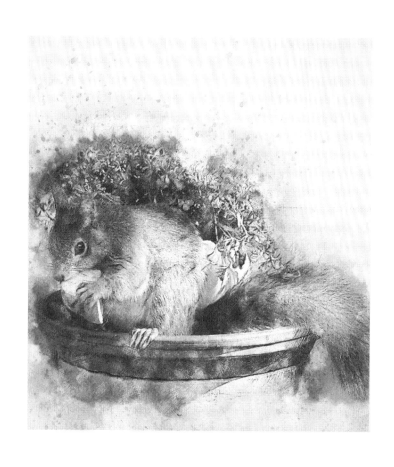

Chapter 4
Apple Cider Vinegar for Pets

"Until one has loved an animal
A part of one's soul remains unawakened."
Anatole France

Dogs!

As apple cider vinegar is a natural product derived from apples, it's safe for dogs as a remedy for many ailments and is certainly a pre-
ferred substitute for chemical-based products, as it has
no artificial ingredients and no harsh chemicals.

According to *Whole Dog Journal*, apple cider vinegar
for dogs is healthy and beneficial. Phosphorus, iron,
calcium, potassium, magnesium, and other crucial
minerals and vitamins are natural health boosters.

Fleas, Ticks, Rashes, Infections, Hot Spots
From preventing fleas to treating ear infections, apple
cider vinegar is a helpful supplement for pet owners
who want to avoid chemicals that may negatively af-

fect their beloved pet. It helps relieve itchiness and rashes, and can prevent yeast infections. Its acidic acid helps eliminate dandruff.

Apple cider vinegar is a natural tick and flea repellent by acidifying the dog's pH. Spraying a dog with a fifty-fifty solution of apple cider vinegar and water prevents ticks and fleas from infesting the dog's fur, and also calms itchy, scaly, dry skin. At the same time, it will bring shiny life back to a dog's dull coat and remove stains from saliva-stained fur, giving the dog's coat a beautiful shine.

Harmful viruses and bacteria will not find a home on your dog's body because of apple cider vinegar's natural antiseptic and antibiotic attributes. It's one of the best remedies for supporting a dog's health and natural immunity to hazardous infections.

Holistic veterinarians advise pet owners to use apple cider vinegar for hot spots, also known as acute moist dermatitis, which are painful, red areas of infected, irritated skin that are sometimes raised. Apple cider vinegar can help dry the hot spot out and eliminate the need to shave the dog.

The best way to keep a dog's ears clean and free of bacteria and yeast is to use a topical solution of fifty-fifty of water and apple cider vinegar, with its antibacterial healing strength.

Digestion

Adding a little apple cider vinegar with its powerful enzymes to your dog's drinking water can do wonders in healing diarrhea and constipation, and reducing gas and bloating. You may also notice your dog loses a bit of weight with some apple cider vinegar in the water.

Muscle Sprains, Bruises, Arthritis, & Joint Discomfort

Apple cider vinegar can ease the pain of a dog's bruises, sore muscles, joint inflammation, and arthritis, when applied topically, and a tablespoon of apple cider vinegar to the dog's food two or three times a week will help break down calcium deposits.

Dental Health

Apple cider vinegar is helpful in the prevention of tooth decay, breaking down plaque, and removing tartar from the dog's teeth. A teaspoon of apple cider vinegar added to food or drinking water is good for doggie's oral health.

Preventing or Healing UTIs

If your dog is prone to urinary tract infections (UTIs), the antibacterial and antiseptic qualities of apple cider vinegar are highly effective in preventing, or when necessary, treating, infections.

The recommended dose of apple cider vinegar for dogs is between one and three teaspoons per day, depending on the dog's weight. One teaspoon for a small to medium dog, and up to three teaspoons for a medium to large dog. Start small and gradually increase the dose as the dog becomes adjusted to the remedy.

Do not give your dog too much apple cider vinegar, as it may irritate the eyes, skin, or the digestive tract. When used internally, apple cider vinegar can cause dehydration. Be sure your beloved pet's water bowl is always full.

Cats!

Cats of all ages can get ill or experience issues that hinder their quality of life. Some cats experience the same issues again and again throughout their lives, such as urinary tract infections or upper respiratory infections.

With apple cider vinegar's enzymes, important vitamins and minerals, and gut-friendly bacteria, it can provide powerful holistic healing, promoting healthy digestion, repelling parasites, and even breaking up bladder crystals.

Fight Off a Urinary Tract Infection

Apple cider vinegar is an excellent healing option for kitty's urinary tract infection. It can be used to create proper pH balance in your cat's urine, and to maintain it, which works to get rid of bacteria. Reduced bacteria will allow the cat's urinary tract to heal naturally and stay healthy. You can use apple cider vinegar when infection symptoms arise until they subside, or use it regularly to prevent the onset of future urinary tract problems. Mix half a teaspoon of apple cider vinegar into the cat's water or food.

Healing an Upper Respiratory Infection

Apple cider vinegar can help a cat get rid of an upper respiratory infection. It works as an expectorant to help your cat breathe easier, which should also improve appetite, and increase water consumption, which is especially important while congested.

You can rub a fifty-fifty apple cider vinegar and water solution on Kitty's paws, chest, and even on the back of the neck, which will be ingested during grooming. Be sure to avoid the eyes and nose.

Fleas, Mites, and Flies

Insects dislike the acidity of apple cider vinegar, and it will effectively repel them. When apple cider vinegar is on a cat's coat, pests will avoid her. Make a fifty-fifty apple cider vinegar and water solution and put it in a spray bottle. Spray kitty and rub the mixture into her coat. Spray daily to keep the fleas away.

How Apple Cider Vinegar Benefits Cats

• Boosts the immune system

• Improves skin and coat health: hotspots, dander, itchiness, fleas

• Fights urinary tract infections

• Helps break up bladder and kidney stones

• Improves metabolism

• Heals candida

Improve Heart Health in Pets

Apple cider vinegar improves several of the biological factors linked to a pet's risk factors for heart disease. It lowers cholesterol, triglycerides, and blood pressure, a major risk factor for kidney and heart disease.

Chapter High Points:

1. Apple cider vinegar is safe to use for many ailments your pet may be suffering.

2. Calcium, iron, magnesium, phosphorus, potassium, and other crucial minerals and vitamins in apple cider vinegar are natural health boosters for dogs and cats.

3. Apple cider vinegar acidifies a dog or cat's coat, which is a natural repellent for insects, and makes the coat shiny, too!

4. Apple cider vinegar's enzymes help heal a variety of intestinal issues.

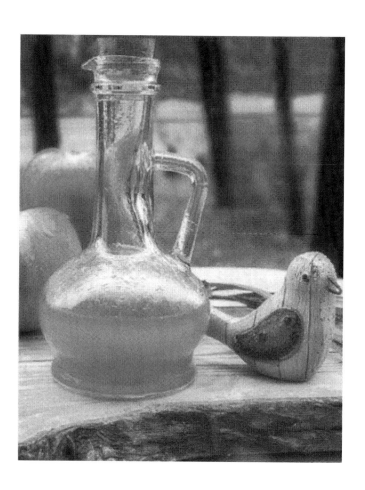

Chapter 5
Apple Cider Vinegar Around the Home

*"The objective of cleaning is not just to clean,
But to feel happiness living within that environment."*
Marie Kondo

Apple Cider Vinegar for a Clean Home
Apple cider vinegar makes a great all-purpose cleaner. Add half a cup to a cup of water in a spray bottle. Use it to clean kitchen counters, windows, appliance surfaces, tile, windows, showers, mirrors, and all other non-porous surfaces.

Clean the toilet with apple cider vinegar by pouring a cup into the bowl and letting it sit overnight. Scrub it clean in the morning!

A tablespoon or two of apple cider vinegar added to the dishwasher makes extra-sparkly disinfected dishes. Apple cider vinegar added to a sink of dishes for hand washing helps break down food residue. Vinegar also kills bacteria and other pathogens.

Apple Cider Vinegar for the Garden

Because of apple cider vinegar's five percent acid content and its nutritional Mother, it can be used to fertilize acid-loving plants such as roses, rhododendrons, lavender, azaleas, blueberry, cranberries, and gardenias. Use an ounce to a gallon solution, and water the plants at their base, as the apple cider vinegar may burn the leaves. Be sure to regularly check the acidity.

Apple cider vinegar also helps the soil release iron, which is beneficial for plants.

Clean Dirty Leaves

With a much more diluted mixture of a teaspoon of apple cider vinegar to a gallon of water, gently wipe off the leaves with a soft cloth. The leaves will shine, and the residual vinegar will deter mites and other pests. Apple cider vinegar also acts as an anti-fungal for happy plants.

Speaking of Pests....

Spray undiluted apple cider vinegar around the circumference of the area where you do not want snails, slugs, rodents, cats, and dogs to enter. The smell is repellent to them. This will need to be done on a weekly basis and after a rainstorm. Be careful not to let overspray contact the plants.

Daily spray ant hills with a fifty-fifty solution of apple cider vinegar until you see the ants have picked up residence and moved.

Clean Rusty Tools

Spray apple cider vinegar on rusty tools and use a scouring pad or steel wool to clean off rust that is beginning to form. If the rust is more deeply set, let the tool/s sit in apple cider vinegar for a day, and then scrub.

Dinner on the Patio

Leave a small container or two of apple cider vinegar on the terrace or patio to alleviate mosquitoes and gnats, as they will be attracted to the vinegar, clearing the air, at least temporarily, of these insects.

Clean Up the Gifts from Birds

Spray apple cider vinegar on bird droppings and let sit for a few moments. The little gifts will readily wipe up, while, at the same time, the apple cider vinegar kills any germs and bacteria.

Chapter High Points:

1. Apple cider vinegar makes the house spick and span clean, while at the same time disinfecting from bacteria and other pathogens.

2. The Mother and the acid content in apple cider vinegar fertilizes acid-loving plants, releases iron from the soil, and deters mites and other insects.

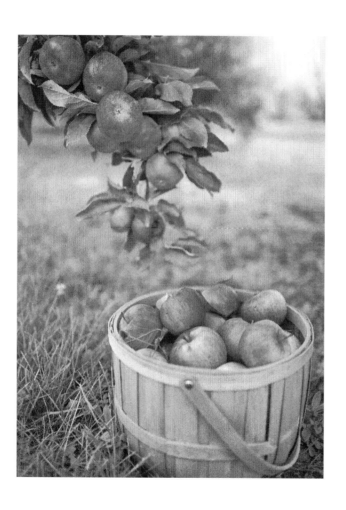

Chapter 6

Apple Cider Vinegar for a Balanced pH

"Keeping your body healthy
is an expression of gratitude
to the whole cosmos."
Thich Nhat Hanh

I s it not frustrating when people—even doctors—get on the internet and on *YouTube,* and start to rant about how unimportant the pH of the body is, because the blood must be slightly alkaline, at a pH between 7.35 and 7.45? And so, they say, it doesn't matter what your diet is, whether acidic or alkaline, because the body will make adjustments for the blood.

Does this make sense? Is it not true that when you put something into a container, that's what comes out? How much more so is the case with our precious bodies?

Yes, the body will make adjustments for blood, because if blood is not between 7.35 and 7.45, slightly alkaline, *the individual dies*. That still doesn't change the fact that the Standard American Diet—appropriately referred to as *SAD*—is acidic and decidedly out of pH balance.

Here is a short list of a few foods and other influences that are acid-forming in the human body:

Dairy

Eggs

Fast food

Fried foods

Packaged foods and additives that preserve packaged food

Caffeinated, carbonated drinks / sodas

Pizza (triple whammy acid-making: wheat crust, dairy cheese, meat)

White sugar

Corn syrup

Artificial sweeteners

Refined salt

Red and Processed Meats. In addition, according to the *American Cancer Society* and *The International Agency for Research on Cancer*, processed and red meats are class one carcinogens.

Seafood

Wheat products (bread, cereals, etc.)

Hectic lifestyle/Stress

Contaminated environment

Health concerns are stressful and thus, acid-forming

This acidic diet is very, *very* hard on your body, which has to work diligently to keep the blood in the required alkaline range. When a body has to maintain the blood's pH with these harmful, acidic, raw materials, it leads to excess weight, fatigue, foggy-mindedness, and life-threatening diseases.

What are some other side effects of an overly acidic diet?

Acid Reflux – A condition in which acid from the stomach flows back up the esophagus causing heartburn and chest pain. Acidic foods contribute to acid reflux by relaxing the esophageal sphincter. Caffeinated drinks, high-fat foods, and alcohol are examples of items that contribute to acid reflux.

Lower Bone Density – overly acidic diet causes an increase in the amount of calcium that a body flushes out, augmenting a higher risk of osteoporosis. A study in the *Journal of Osteoporosis International* from Switzerland showed that the acidic diet of participants increased the amount of calcium flushed out through urine by *seventy-four percent*.

Kidney Stones – Acidic acid increases the risk of uric or cystine kidney stones.

Decrease Hormone Levels –Acidosis can lead to a decrease in levels of the human growth hormone (HGH), produced by the pituitary gland, which is responsible for cell regeneration and growth.

Chronic Pain – Acidic foods cause inflammation which contributes to chronic systemic pain, chronic back pain, muscle spasms, and headaches.

And the list goes on.

It would be cause for celebration if the people who broadcast their errors regarding pH balance came to know the actual science of how body chemistry works, and stopped preaching this incorrect information, encouraging people to continue with their horrible diet.

Check out the diets of the Blue Zones on earth, where people live the longest—and more importantly—the healthiest! with alkaline-based diet: Loma Linda, CA, Nicoya, Costa Rica, Sardinia, Italy, Ikaria, Greece, Okinawa, Japan.

It's true that apple cider vinegar can work to improve your pH balance. But why make it work so hard peddling uphill, in an effort to bring the body into an average healthy pH balance, when if your diet was already pH balanced, apple cider vinegar could work to augment your health and longevity into excellence?

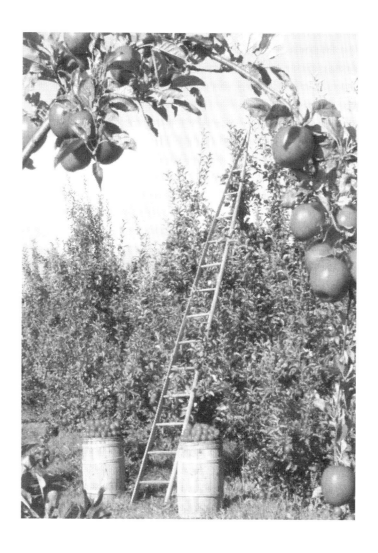

Chapter 7
How to Make the Mother
& Apple Cider Vinegar Recipes

"The greatest wealth is health."
Ralph Waldo Emerson

T he Process of Making the Mother

An apple cider vinegar Mother, or SCOBY; "a symbiotic culture of bacteria and yeast," is a gelatinous biofilm that forms on the top of the apple cider being made into vinegar. It's a form of cellulose that manifests from the natural bacteria that produce acetic acid, a core element of all vinegar.

The ever-present bacteria in the air convert the alcohol in cider into acetic acid, giving vinegar its sharp, sour taste. That is to say, the bacteria that makes vinegar feeds on the alcohol of the apple cider, and in the process creates acetic acid and the film of cellulose called the Mother.

Exposure To Air

As the Mother forms on the surface of the alcohol it is fermenting, it needs to have maximum exposure to oxygen, wherein resides the natural bacteria. Use a plain glass, wide-mouthed, jar for this process. Do not use ceramic, crystal glass, or metal containers.

To stop little creatures and dust from entering and ruining the vinegar fermentation, cover the opening with cheesecloth or even a couple of layers of paper towel and secure it with a rubber band or string. Be sure that whatever you use to cover the jar is both dense enough to not allow even the tiniest bug or dust to enter, while permitting the air to freely flow.

Once you have a Mother, you can then produce other batches of apple cider vinegar with it, transferring the bulk of the Mother to the new batch, while leaving some of its health-making threads in the original batch of apple cider vinegar.

Details of Making the Mother from Scratch

Again, be sure not to use any metal pans, pots, or spoons in the process.

Choose your apples. Any apple will do, but a suggestion is to use two sweet apples to one tart apple for a complex flavor.

Wash and cut each apple into cubes. Include the cores and seeds—no need to get overly fussy. Just throw it all in.

Cover with filtered water, free from impurities. Any apple not entirely covered by the water will rot and ruin the vinegar. If they poke out of the water, cover with something that is not metal, to keep them submerged.

Add one heaping teaspoon of sugar per apple (raw sugar is best, but any will do). Stir thoroughly. It's the sugar that ferments and turns into alcohol.

Cover the jar with cheesecloth, a coffee filter, or some other breathable material that fruit flies cannot get through, and secure it with a rubber band.

Keep the jar in a warm, dark, undisturbed location.

Stir a bit every day or two, to make sure the apples are submerged.

In a week or two, you'll see bubbles in the jar, which indicate that fermentation is in process. When the apples sink to the bottom of the jar, they have fermented and are no longer needed.

Strain the cider through the cheesecloth, set aside the apples, and return the cider to the jar. Cover again with cheesecloth, put it back in its warm, dark place, and leave it to ferment for several weeks to, perhaps, months. Making vinegar is somewhat more an art than a science.

Test the acid content, which should be about four percent. You can purchase an acid testing kit from a winemaking shop or online for fifty to one-hundred dollars … or you can use pH strips purchased from your local pharmacy, or online, for a few dollars. Dip the strip in the vinegar and its color will let you know its acidity. The strips come with their own specific directions for you to follow.

The longer you let the apple cider vinegar ferment, the stronger it will be. During this time, if you're fortunate, the Mother, a gelatinous cellulose thick film, will form on the surface.

Use this precious Mother to produce more vinegar.

If this all seems a bit arduous and time-consuming, you can jump-start the process by buying acid cider vinegar that has the Mother, and add that to your vinegar-making process. Use it in place of some of the water, perhaps about a third. Again, making vinegar is more an art than a science.

Enjoy making art!

Purchasing an Apple Cider Vinegar Mother
Another option is to purchase an apple cider vinegar Mother/SCOBY. Here are a few resources. I'm sure there are many others. I'd be interested to hear about your experience with any of these, or others, you may discover.

Olivewood Brewing & Craft Company
https://www.olivewoodbrewing.com/search?type=product&q=apple+cider+vinegar+mother

Hobby Home Brew
https://www.hobbyhomebrew.com/product/mother-of-vinegar-for-apple-cider-vinegar-by-supreme-8oz-236-ml/

F.H. Steinbart
https://fhsteinbart.com/product/supremeapple-cidervinegarmother/

Supreme Vinegar
https://www.amazon.com/Supreme-Cider-Mother-of-Vinegar/dp/B00NRBGIUK

Southern Home Brew
https://southernhomebrew.com/applevinegar.html

A Few Apple Cider Vinegar Recipes

There are so many things that can be done with apple cider vinegar. Following are just a few recipes that will perhaps get your curiosity in motion about what else might be done with apple cider vinegar. Thousands of recipes can be found on the internet that explores its wonders.

Perhaps you'll even come up with a recipe of your own. If you do, I'd love to see it!

Here's a recipe for a super-healing concoction that can have a positive effect on everything from acne to arthritis. Or take a daily dose as a general health and fitness tonic.

Super Apple Cider Vinegar

Put one cup of apple cider vinegar, one cup of honey (Manuka honey is even better), and 10 peeled cloves of garlic in a blender.

Mix on high speed until well blended. Pour the mixture into a glass container. Seal and keep in the refrigerator. Take one teaspoon to one tablespoon in a glass of water or fruit juice, from one to three times daily, as suits your own constitution.

Ginger Apple Cider Vinegar Whammy!

Ginger is closely related to turmeric and, like apple cider vinegar, has anti-inflammatory, antioxidant, and free radical benefits. Adding ginger to apple cider vinegar multiplies the potential.

One tablespoon apple cider vinegar

One tablespoon ginger, either the ground spice, or for more benefit, grate fresh ginger

One tablespoon of healthy sweetener, such as maple syrup, monk fruit, honey, or xylitol

Two cups water and ice

Stir together and enjoy the refreshing, power-packed beverage.

Hot, Hot Apple Cider Vinegar Beverage

Try this warm-you-up beverage on a chilly day—or just when you feel like a toasty drink! Cinnamon is also full of antioxidants and works to lower blood sugar. Cayenne pepper contains minerals and vitamins that boost metabolism through thermogenesis, an increase in the body's heat that *burns calories*.

One tablespoon of apple cider vinegar

One-quarter teaspoon ground cinnamon, either ground spice, or grate fresh cinnamon

One tablespoon of your favorite, healthy sweetener

A dash or two of cayenne pepper (to taste!)

Stir together in a cup of hot water.

Apple Cider Vinegar Yummy Purple Potato Salad

Purple potatoes are not only pretty, but their color lets us know that they are rich in polyphenyl antioxidants called anthocyanins, also found in blackberries and blueberries. *Yay for the purple family!*

Anthocyanins contribute to healthy levels of cholesterol, reduced risk of diabetes and heart disease, plus improved vision and healthy eyes. Purple potatoes have two-to-three times more antioxidant power than white or yellow potatoes!

Ingredients:
Two pounds of purple potatoes
Half-a-cup of green onions
One-third cup sweet relish

Dressing:
One-half cup veganaise or mayonnaise
One tablespoon of your favorite mustard (I like honey mustard)
One tablespoon apple cider vinegar
Dash of salt & pepper

Place potatoes in a pot and cover with water. Add a pinch of salt
Bring to a boil, cook for fifteen minutes on gentle boil, until potatoes are tender but still firm
Drain and cool
Cut potatoes into cubes

While potatoes are cooking, combine the dressing ingredients in a bowl and stir. Add a bit of water if consistency is too thick for your preference.

Pour potatoes into a large salad bowl, add the onions, stir.

Add the dressing and mix.

Season with salt and pepper to taste.

Apple Cider Vinegar Shell Pasta Salad

One pound shell pasta or gluten-free shell pasta

One-half red onion, diced

One red or yellow bell pepper, diced

Half-a-cup walnuts, or other favorite nuts

2 cups frozen or fresh peas

Dressing:

One cup veganaise or mayonnaise

One-quarter cup apple cider vinegar

One tablespoon of your favorite mustard

One tablespoon maple syrup

Dash of salt & pepper

Boil shell paste until it is al dente, drain under cool water.

Combine the dressing ingredients in a small bowl, whisking until creamy.

Add the shell pasta, red onion, bell pepper nuts and peas in a large bowl.

Add the dressing and mix together.

Season with salt and pepper to taste.

Apple Cider Vinegar Divine Cornbread

One cup of yellow cornmeal
One cup spelt flour
One tablespoon baking powder
One-third cup organic sugar
One cup almond or oat milk
One-third cup light-flavored olive oil
One-quarter teaspoon salt
Two tablespoons apple cider vinegar

Preheat oven to four hundred degrees.
Lightly grease 8-inch square pan, or line with parchment paper.
Mixed together milk, sugar, oil, and apple cider vinegar
In another bowl, add the cornmeal, flour, baking powder, and salt.
Whisk these ingredients together.
Pour the wet ingredients into the dry ingredients and whip lightly.

Pour the batter into the pan and bake for 25 minutes, or until golden brown and a toothpick comes out clean.

Enjoy with your favorite fruit preserves, or as a tasty addition to dinner.

Yummy, Super Easy Black Bean Soup

Two cans of black beans

One large onion, chopped
Four cloves of garlic, chopped
One red bell pepper, chopped
One teaspoon cumin
Two cups of vegetable broth
One bay leaf, optional
One-quarter cup apple cider vinegar
Dash of salt & pepper

Drain and rinse the black beans, add all the ingredients except the apple cider vinegar into a pot, and bring to a boil.
Reduce heat and simmer for twenty minutes.
Alternatively, you may wish to sauté the onions and pepper, then add them to the soup.
After removing the soup from the stove, add the apple cider vinegar, and stir.
Garnish with chopped Roma tomatoes and onion.

Beautiful! Delish! And so good for you!

Root for Apple Cider Vinegar & Root Veggies!

Root vegetables are fantastic. They keep well if stored properly. Because they grow under the ground, they have an abundance of nutrients and minerals from the soil. They are wonderfully filling, and super healthy!

Two sweet potatoes
Two parsnips
Two carrots

Two rutabagas
One red onion
One tablespoon of your favorite mustard
Three tablespoons extra-virgin olive oil
One teaspoon dried thyme
one-quarter cup apple cider vinegar
One-to-two teaspoons salt

Preheat oven to 450°
Cut all the vegetables into long wedges or thick slices.
Combine all the ingredients in a large bowl then add the vegetables and coat them evenly.
Line a baking sheet with parchment paper, and spread the vegetables in a single layer.
Bake for 30 minutes, or until the vegetables are evenly roasted.

Do you have someone in your life who thinks they don't like vegetables? See if roasted root veggies, with the zing of apple cider vinegar and mustard will change their mind!

Sweet Treat Lemon Cake
One cup almond, soy, or oat milk
One cup +two tablespoons of flour or gluten-free flour
One teaspoon apple cider vinegar
One-third cup ground almonds
One and one-half teaspoon baking powder
One-half teaspoon salt
One cup organic sugar

One-third cup of your favorite plant-based oil
Juice from one small lemon
Two tablespoons lemon zest

Icing:
One-half cup powdered sugar
One tablespoon almond, soy, or oat milk
Two teaspoons lemon juice or one-half teaspoon lemon extract

Preheat oven to 350°
Line a loaf pan with parchment paper, or lightly spray with oil.
Stir together the milk and apple cider vinegar in a medium bowl.
In a large bowl mix together the flour, almond meal, baking powder and salt.
In the medium bowl add to the milk and vinegar the sugar, oil, lemon juice, lemon zest, and stir well.
Pour the wet ingredients into the dry ingredients and stir until combined. Do not over stir.
Pour the batter into the pan. Bake for thirty-five to forty minutes, or until a toothpick inserted comes out clean.
When through baking, let it sit for ten minutes until it cools, before removing from the pan.
Whisk together the icing ingredients. Once the cake is completely cool, drizzle the icing on top.
An elegant cake with *both* lemon and apple cider vinegar … it just doesn't get any better!

Switchel

Way back at the beginning of the book when I was sharing a bit about apple cider vinegar's long and prodigious history, I mentioned Ruth of the Bible, who was working in the fields when Boaz, whom she subsequently married, who invited her to share some bread dipped in vinegar.

That tradition has carried on through the ages. Hippocrates wrote of a vinegar and honey beverage called, "oxymel."

And in our own times, we have "switchel," a mixture of water, apple cider vinegar, local sweetener, spiced with ginger.

Popular in the American Colonies

Switchel became popular in the American colonies by the late 1600s. This came about because of the availability of Caribbean ingredients such as molasses and ginger. The proportions of the ingredients, and the ingredients themselves, changed according to individual tastes and local ingredients. For example, in New England they used maple syrup, and in the southern states, sorghum was common. But the core ingredient has always been apple cider vinegar.

Switchel was a common staple by the 1800s throughout the United States. It was even referred to in *Little House on the Prairie*, the stories by Laura Ingalls Wilder. A mixture of water, sugar, vinegar, and ginger was carried out to the fields to refresh the family, harvesting hay in the summer heat.

Haymaker's Punch

Switchel became so common, that it was called, "haymaker's punch" by the farming community. The reason it became so popular is because it brings about rapid hydration, and replaces electrolytes.

Long before people understood the notion of electrolytes, they clearly understood the rejuvenating and healing nature of apple cider vinegar in water with a bit of sweetness. The potassium helps replenish the body after hard work, and the ginger soothes the digestive system, with all the components contributing to help reduce inflammation and sore muscles.

It's the combination of sweet and tangy that's so refreshing. The farming crews would take a jug of switchel and place it in a stream or spring if they were lucky enough to have one nearby, or under a shade tree to keep it cool.

Now, as then, it remains a rejuvenating and refreshing beverage. Ground ginger is fine, but you can't beat freshly grated ginger, with its invigorating flavor. Sweetener of choice still remains a mainstay of switchel, but the natural syrups of maple or molasses, or honey, offer the most health benefits.

You may discover that you love to take your home-made switchel with you when you go to the gym!

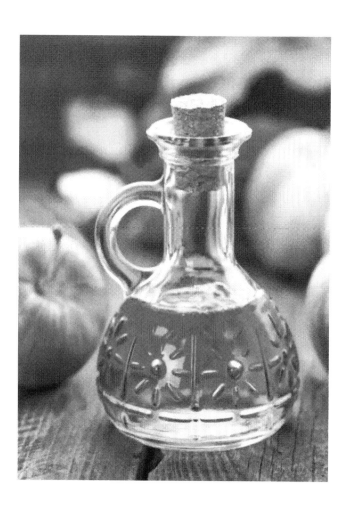

Chapter 8
Brands of Apple Cider Vinegar

"Physical fitness is not only one of the most important keys to a healthy body, it is the basis of dynamic and creative intellectual activity."
John F. Kennedy

Here are a few brands of apple cider vinegar with the Mother. Bragg is referred to and lauded far and wide, and it's great. But there are others, and I encourage users to try different brands. As the making of apple cider vinegar is, as previously mentioned, an art more than a science, you may discover that some other brand is particularly suitable for your body and taste.

Recall that the product is a result of different apples, fermented at different seasons, in different environments, with different attendant bacteria. Keep in mind that ingesting products that are native to one's own territory often have superior benefit.

Dynamic Health Organic Raw Apple Cider Vinegar with Mother

Eden Foods Organic Apple Cider Vinegar with Mother

Vitacost Certified Organic Apple Cider Vinegar with Mother

Bragg Organic Raw Unfiltered Apple Cider Vinegar with Mother

Spectrum Organic Apple Cider Vinegar with Mother

Simple Truth Raw Unfiltered Apple Cider Vinegar With Mother

Sanniti Organic Apple Cider Vinegar Unfiltered with the Mother

Swanson Certified Organic Apple Cider Vinegar with Mother

There are others, but if they don't specifically say "with the Mother" on the packaging, I've not included them. I'm sure there are many others that I haven't encountered in my research, not to mention that there are no doubt wonderful apple cider vinegars in remote parts of the world that we all wish we could enjoy!

Also, in my extensive research, I've encountered numerous personal reports that the capsule form is not as effective as the liquid apple cider vinegar, with quite a few people saying it doesn't work at all. I, personally, stick with glass-bottled liquid, so I haven't addressed any other form. However, I'm always open to any and all comments, testimonials, or reviews regarding apple cider vinegar that you might want to share.

"I meant to do my work today
But a brown bird sang in the apple tree
And a butterfly flitted across the field
And all the leaves were calling me."
Richard Le Gallienne

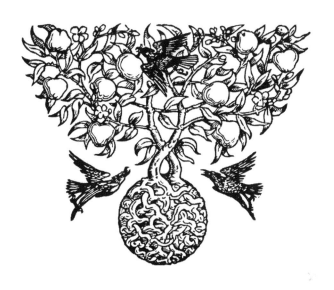

"The goldenrod is yellow,
The corn is turning brown,
The trees in apple orchards
With fruit are bending down."
Helen Hunt Jackson

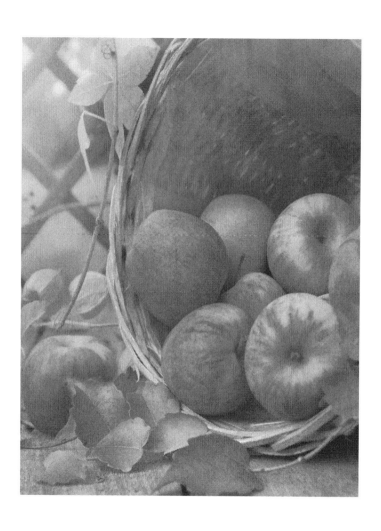

Chapter 9
Apple Cider Vinegar Testimonials

"To avoid sickness eat less,
To prolong life worry less."
Chu Hui Weng

H eartburn
Connie – Eugene, Oregon
"I recommend anyone with heartburn to keep ACV with cloves of garlic in the refrigerator and drink an ounce of that mixture next time heartburn occurs. The result is almost immediate."

Ray – New York City
"I used to get severe heartburn after eating spicy things. A friend recommended I drink a tablespoon of apple cider vinegar. In less than a minute the burning sensations were gone!"

Anonymous
"I used to suffer from heartburn after every meal. Even after breakfast! After stumbling on ACV, I have not suffered from heartburn ever since. It has cured my sinus

headaches and a wart that I had on my finger for five years went away!"

Acid Reflux
Rasheeda – Arlington, TX

"I had a very bad case of acid reflux. No over the counter medicine worked. I then remembered an article I read that apple cider vinegar cures acid reflux. I took two table-spoons 3 times that day and the acid reflux went away."

Acid Reflux
Larry – Bellwood, Illinois

"Recently, I started taking a tablespoon of apple cider vinegar twice a day to help with my life long acid reflux. I'd heard that my medication was stopping my natural production of stomach acid, and that the apple cider vinegar would supply me with the natural amounts needed for proper digestion. I have now been two weeks free without my OTC meds. I have never felt better, and I am not afraid to go to bed without my OTC meds."

Rheumatoid Arthritis
Anonymous

"This has been helpful with my RA and digestion. Still new to this treatment, but certainly has shown a differ-ence in my RA pain. Praying it lasts."

Kidney Stones
Dave

"The reason I first took ACV is I had heard it was good for kidney stones. Three days after starting with it the stone that was painful was gone. I did not pass it, it just vanished. Since I am also diabetic, I noticed my blood sugar levels were lower so I continue taking it."

Horse has no More Colic
Isabel – France
"My mare had a tendency to have colic due to obstructions as well as spasmodic colic. But this is no longer the case thanks to apple cider vinegar!"

Cure for Hand Cramps
Masterchief – Lawrenceburg, Ky
"After being told to drink more water, take vitamins, stretch and massage my hand, nothing worked to relieve my painful hand cramps and sometimes leg cramps. But I recently tried apple cider vinegar, honey and water. In about two minutes my hand cramps were gone!"

Blood Sugar
Robert – Mississippi
"Been using ACV for about two months, great results with sugar numbers. Dropped from 127 to as low as 83. I Take ACV just before meals. At age 73 I do not take any prescription medicine and don't intend to.

"I've been pre-diabetic for eight years. My numbers went over the line to 7.0 for the first time. That is when I read about ACV. While taking ACV I have also lost ten pounds, I have more energy, no more occasional blurry vision, and I sleep better. Hope ACV works so well for you also."

Chronic Fatigue
Anonymous

"A few weeks ago I looked up potential remedies that said apple cider vinegar cures chronic fatigue. It said the acetic acid in apple cider vinegar is part of the citric acid cycle of the human body and that vinegar is not acid-forming in the body, contrary to what I'd read some years ago elsewhere. It said the fatigue should end in about two hours after trying vinegar.

"So I got some apple cider vinegar that day and tried some with my food. And two hours later I felt significantly energized, as promised. The next day I was able to ride my bike nine miles each way on a hilly road to the farm, where I worked for several hours hoeing around my Kiefer pear trees. Now it's been several weeks and I have several tablespoons of vinegar a day and my energy level has been very good. I rode the bike to the farm two days this week to pick pears and make pear juice with my brother's cider press, as I want to make vinegar from the juice."

No More Inhaler!
Robert – Clarkston, MI

"I have been using the apple cider vinegar and honey treatment for 3 days now and last night was the first time, during my martial arts class, that i was able to make it all the way through the class without using an inhaler. The inhaler didn't always work. my lungs didn't become restricted while breathing heavy and i was able to take normal breaths while running. i am amazed at the effectiveness of this natural cure and have already passed it on to family and friends. it is working great for me so far and i will continue to take it. i will not be using my inhaler anymore."

Asthma & Sinus Problems
Jean – Upper Marlboro, MD

"I am taking apple cider vinegar for asthma & sinus problems. Also using it for weight loss, just found that out today. I was glad to try an over-the-counter remedy for my ailments. I hate using prescribed medicine because they don't resolve the problem, instead it just makes it worse.

"I have been health conscious since I was sixteen, and surprised when my doctor told me I had developed asthma; which he stated was triggered by my allergies. Before I found your site I had been using A vitamin, NAC, Quercetin, fish oil, etc., to keep my asthma at bay; but I had two asthma attacks in April, when everything started blooming. I didn't want to take steroids, so I went on the internet, since I wanted to do it naturally and not by a prescription.

"I am very happy to say that apple cider vinegar has worked for me. I take two tablespoons a day straight up. It has also helped with my sinus problem, and allergies. I love it, and just to think I had the cure for my asthma in my cupboard all that time and didn't know it. I'm also going to try the other remedies for losing weight."

Asthma
Katherine – Las Vegas, Nevada
"Two tablespoons of apple cider vinegar in a glass of water cured tightness in my chest and throat due to asthma. When visiting my boyfriend in Connecticut, I had an asthma attack and didn't have my inhaler. After I regained my breath I drank this mixture and almost instantaneously the tightness in my chest and throat relaxed and the wheezing, uncomfortable breathing, stopped."

Hand Cramps
Anonymous – Pennsylvania
"I have had very, very, severe pain with hand cramps which became increasingly worse over the last several years.

"I used every kind of prescription medication my doctor recommended with no benefit. On the last prescription trial of sixty days, with constant pain and cramping, I had no relief, whatsoever.

"I turned to the internet out of desperation and found apple cider vinegar recommended. I took two teaspoons in eight ounces of water with one teaspoon of honey as suggested.

"To repeat, before taking this I was in pain for years. Without any exaggeration, in less than two minutes my pain was gone, and I haven't had any pain, for over three months. Apple cider vinegar is like a miracle. This is unbelievable but true!"

Heat Exhaustion
Anonymous

"I have always struggled with heat and outdoor activities, but recently I experienced a case of full blown heat exhaustion: chills, headache, nausea, heartburn and fatigue. I could do absolutely nothing but lie in bed propped up. I tried taking 1 Tablespoon ACV in a glass of water. I did not think I could get it down, but I did. This helped calm my nausea and heartburn, and allowed me to drift into sleep.

"The next morning, I felt eighty percent better, and was so grateful to have no more nausea. After speaking with a doctor about this experience, I was told that once you experience a case of heat stress you are more vulnerable to repeat cases until your body fully heals. This was indeed my situation—I had had a similar experience three weeks prior. It is good to know that the body takes its time to heal from these events, and I will give myself more time before tackling another challenging exposed hike."

Arthritis
Lisa

"My sister absolutely swears by this stuff! She doesn't have arthritis in her hands anymore, thanks to her daily glass of water with apple cider vinegar."

Tastes Great & I'm Feeling Better
Rhonda

"Before I gave it a try, I used to believe ACV surely would have to be one of the worst-tasting things around. To my surprise, I actually LIKE it. Really. If you mix a teaspoon or two of it in a glass of water and stir in a teaspoon of honey (to taste), you'll find that it tastes a lot like lemonade. Then when you start feeling better, you'll not want to give it up! It can actually stop certain allergic reactions in a matter of minutes."

Gout is Gone!
Doug – Michigan, United States
"ACV is nothing short of a miracle....

"A teaspoon in the morning, a teaspoon in the evening. Day one: slight reduction in swelling. Day two: not much change. Day three: Gout is completely gone, and I mean completely! No swelling, no pain. This is the best stuff on the planet for gout, and for your health in general.

"P.S. apple cider vinegar must contain the *Mother* to work its magic."

Helps With Arthritic Pain
Shell – UK
"I was looking for a natural probiotic to take after being on back-to-back antibiotics. A friend recommended apple cider vinegar with Mother and added that it may also help with my arthritic pain. I started drinking one table-

spoon of apple cider vinegar in a cup of water and just after three days, I felt the improvement in my gut and my finger joints.

"I'm now taking two tablespoons of apple cider per cup of water. You feel that your tummy is being "cleaned". I also noticed that my hands are no longer stiff and in pain when I wake up in the morning. Really pleased with the result. I will continue drinking apple cider vinegar with the Mother to put good bacteria back in my gut and as an anti-inflammatory. Highly Recommended!"

Heartburn/Acid Reflux
James Murphy
"I use apple cider vinegar twice a day. I started because it was a natural treatment for heartburn and acid reflux and it worked like a charm. I feel a lot better when I'm taking it twice a day than when I'm not. When I first started, I used to mix it with hot water and honey but once you get used to it you can hit it straight. An essential product in my pantry."

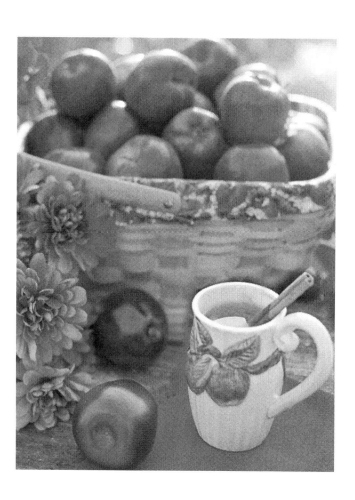

Chapter 10
Apple Cider Vinegar In-Depth Research & Notes

"Happiness is the highest form of health."
Dalai Lama

I have included here some of the research referred to in the book in greater depth, for those of you interested in reading more of the science.

Antimicrobial Activity of Apple Cider Vinegar against Escherichia coli, Staphylococcus aureus and Candida albicans; Downregulating Cytokine and Microbial Protein Expression
https://www.ncbi.nlm.nih.gov/pmc/articles/PMC5788933/
"ACV consists of acetic acid, flavonoids such as gallic acid, tyrosol catechin, epicatechin, benzoic acid, vaninilin, caftaric acid, coutaric acid, caffeic acid, and ferrulic acid. These constituents have been reported to (positively) affect immune defence and oxidative responses.

"Furthermore, the mechanism of ACV activity could be attributed in part to the apple polyphenol content.

Yang *et al.* (2010) reported on the cellular protective effects of apple polyphenols on induced liver damage whereby histopathological tissue destruction was limited and liver activity maintained in mice that received the polyphenols. The mechanisms involved were free radical scavenger action, lipid peroxidation modulation and the antioxidant upregulation capacity of ACV."

"Another reason raw apple cider vinegar may be so beneficial is its mineral content. Apple cider vinegar is rich in calcium, chlorine, copper, iron, magnesium, phosphorous, potassium, silicon, sulfur and other minerals in trace amounts. Apple cider vinegar is best known for its potassium content, which many people are deficient in and is a powerful agent against high blood pressure. For vitamins, apple cider vinegar is a source of Vitamin A, Vitamin B1, Vitamin B2, Vitamin B6, Vitamin C, Vitamin E, beta-carotene, and Vitamin P. It is also rich in pectin.

"Apple cider vinegar is stored as glycerin in the body, which scrubs fat from the cells. It also speeds up the metabolism and accelerates the oxidation process required to flush fats out of the system. The potassium then does a great of job reducing water retention in the body."

Digestive Enzymes
International Journal of Pharmacology
In a rat experiment, after four weeks of apple cider vinegar the rats had a decrease in the digestive components

of maltese, sucrase, and lactase. By decreasing these digestive components, we are decreasing the hydrolysis of a disaccharide to a monosaccharide. And by decreasing these enzymes, the amount of carbohydrates that break down into simple sugars are decreased, which are the simple sugars for the body to absorb.

Free Fatty Acid Receptor
Journal of Diabetes
A study with mice found that acidic acid combined to free fatty acid receptors 2 and 3 triggered a release of glucagon-like peptide 1 and peptide yy. Glucagon peptide 1 slows down gastric emptying, with the result of the food staying in the stomach, resulting in feeling satiated longer. Also, food that digests slower triggers less of a blood sugar spike, and less of a blood sugar drop.

Acidic Acid Activates Hepatic AMPK
& Reduces Hyperglycemia in Diabetic KK-A (y) Mice
Biochemistry and Biophysical Research Communications
In an in vitro study with rat hepatocytes, rat liver cells, the cells were treated with acidic acid. In an hour there was a forty percent increase in the phosphorylation of the energy sensor AMPK, to release fats and carbs.

This may be affected by better glucose utilization in the periphery, through a nitric oxide pathway, cells in our periphery tissues can actually use glucose better, going into the cells in the body and sucking up more glucose.

The liver then directs the liberation of glucose. Secondly, it may inhibit hepatic glucogenic gene expression. At the liver there is less expression of the genes that allow for more gluconeogenesis. There could be a modulation of gluconeogenesis occurring there, which means the liver is releasing fewer carbohydrates.

Examination of the Antiglycemic Properties of Vinegar in Healthy Adults
https://pubmed.ncbi.nlm.nih.gov/20068289/

Vinegar reduces postprandial glycemia (PPG) in healthy adults. This study investigated the vinegar dosage (ten versus twenty grams), timing (during mealtime versus five hours before meal) and application (acetic acid as vinegar vs. neutralized salt) for reducing PPG.

Method

Four randomized crossover trials were conducted in adults (n = 9-10/trial) with type 2 diabetes (one trial) or without diabetes (three trials). All trials followed the same protocol: a standardized meal the evening prior to testing, an overnight fast (one ten hour) and two-hour glucose testing following consumption of a bagel and juice test meal (three trials) or dextrose solution (one trial). For each trial, PPG was compared between treatments using area-under-the-curve calculations one-hundred-twenty minutes after the meal.

Results

Two teaspoons of vinegar (ten grams) effectively reduced PPG, and this effect was most pronounced when vinegar was ingested during mealtime as compared to five hours before the meal. Vinegar did not alter PPG when ingested with monosaccharides, suggesting that the antiglycemic action of vinegar is related to the digestion of carbohydrates. Finally, sodium acetate did not alter PPG, indicating that acetate salts lack antiglycemic properties.

Conclusions

The antiglycemic properties of vinegar are evident when small amounts of vinegar are ingested with meals composed of complex carbohydrates. In these situations, vinegar attenuated PPG by twenty percent compared to placebo.

In Closing ....

I hope you've found *Save Your Life with Awesome Apple Cider Vinegar* useful.

I'm grateful for all the research that has been done investigating apple cider vinegar, providing a wealth of material for me to delve into to write this book. In my extensive research, I was surprised to again and again and *again* read some permutation of the sentence, "There has not been any research to support these claims about apple cider vinegar."

There has been *an abundance of research*. Nor can the many thousands upon thousands of personal testimonials, reports, accounts, descriptions, narratives, and vignettes be readily ignored.

Apple cider vinegar is one of Nature's superlative ways of helping us take care of ourselves. All we need do is to put it to good use in the many ways it can play a part in the cleanliness, health, and well-being of our lives, our children, our pets, and our homes.

Eat Wisely
Exercise Joyfully
Sl-e-e-e-e-p Peacefully ...
Nighty-nite!

Medical Disclaimer

Although this book is based on recent scientific research, the content should not be considered as medical advice or a recommendation for medical treatment. This content is strictly educational and infor-
mational. Readers are strongly recommended to con-
sult with their healthcare professional regarding
health issues and treatments.

Further, there's some evidence that apple cider vinegar may interact with certain drugs. If you take any of
the following medications, please talk with your
health care professional before consuming apple cider
vinegar: digoxin, insulin, diabetes drugs, or diuretics.

My Gift for You ....

As a thank you for reading *Save Your Life with Awesome Apple Cider Vinegar*, I have a gift for you, *Save Your Life with Stupendous Spices*. To receive your ebook, type in the following link:

<u>https://BookHip.com/DKHVDA</u>

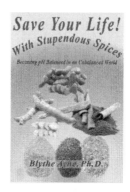

About the Author ....

I live in the midst (and often the mist) of ten acres of forest, with domestic and wild creatures, where I create an ever-growing inventory of self-help, health, and meditation nonfiction books, fiction, short stories, and illustrated kid's books, along with quite a bit of poetry. I've also begun audio recording my books.

I do a bit of wood carving when I need a change of pace, and I'm frequently on a ladder, cleaning my gutters. It's spectacular being on a ladder ... the vista opens up all around, and I feel rather like a bird or a squirrel, perched on a metal branch.

After I received my Doctorate from the University of California at Irvine in the School of Social Sciences, (majoring in psychology and ethnography), I moved to the Pacific Northwest to write and to have a modest private psychotherapy practice in a small town not much bigger than a village.

Finally, I decided it was time to put my full focus on my writing, where, through the world-shrinking internet, I could "meet" greater numbers of people. *Where I could meet you!*

All the creatures in my forest and I are glad you "stopped by." If you enjoyed **Save Your Life with Awesome Apple Cider Vinegar**, I hope you'll share the book with others. If you want to write to me, I'd love to hear from you.

Here's my email:

Blythe@BlytheAyne.com

And here's my website:

www.BlytheAyne.com

And my *Boutique of Books*:

https://shop.BlytheAyne.com

I hope to "see" you again!

Blythe

GLOSSARY:

Acetylcholine - A neuro-transmitting compound found throughout the nervous system.

Acidic - pH below 7.

Albedo - The white pith of citrus fruit.

Alkaline - pH greater than 7.

Allergens - Substances causing allergic reactions.

Antibiotic - A substance that inhibits the growth of or destroys microorganisms.

Antibodies - Blood proteins that combine with substances the body recognizes as alien such as bacteria, viruses, and foreign substances in the blood to destroy them.

Antibacterial - A substance or process that is active against bacteria.

Anti-fungal - A substance or process that is active against fungus.

Antihistamine - A compound for treating allergies that inhibits the effects of histamine.

Anti-inflammatory - Used to reduce inflammation.

Antioxidants - A substance such as vitamin C or E that removes potentially damaging oxidizing agents in a living organism.

Antiseptic - Substances that prevent the growth of disease-causing microorganisms.

Antiviral - A substance or process that is effective against viruses

Apo B - The structural protein of the LDL cholesterol molecule.

Ayurvedic/Ayurveda - East Indian ancient and present-day medicine.

Bile - A bitter greenish-brown alkaline fluid that aids digestion. It is secreted by the liver and stored in the gallbladder.

Bioavailable - A substance that enters circulation when introduced into the body and is able to have an active effect.

Biosynthesis - The production of complex molecules in living organisms or cells.

Calorie - The food calorie (as distinguished from the chemistry calorie, which is one-tenth as much) is the energy needed to raise the temperature of one kilogram of water by one degree Celsius.

Carbohydrates - Organic compounds which include sugars, starch, and cellulose. They contain hydrogen and oxygen in the same ratio as water (2:1) and can be broken down to release energy in the body.

Carcinogenic - Having the potential to cause cancer.

Catalyst - A substance that increases the rate of a chemical reaction without itself changing.

Chelator - A molecule that binds to another, usually larger, molecule.

Cholesterol - A sterol compound found in most body tissues including blood and nerves. Cholesterol and its derivatives are important components of cell membranes.

> **HDL** - good - high-density lipoprotein that removes cholesterol from the blood. It is associated with a reduced risk of atherosclerosis and heart disease.

> **LDL** - bad - the form of lipoprotein in which cholesterol is transported in the blood.

Citric Acid - The primary carrier of biochemicals in the body.

Dietary Fiber - Substances such as cellulose, lignin (organic polymer in many plant cell walls), and pectin, resistant to the action of digestive enzymes.

Electrolytes - The ionized or ionizable components of blood, a living cell, or other organic matter.

Enzymes - Catalysts to specific biochemical reactions. Most enzymes are proteins of large, complex molecules.

Flavonoids - Antioxidant, anti-inflammatory, antimicrobial, anticancer, antibacterial, antibiotic, microbial and anti-fungal, with analgesic, and antiallergic properties plant pigment crystalline compounds. Stops cell division in many cancer cell lines, enhances the functions of vitamin C.

Free Radicals - An unstable molecule missing an electron. They attack stable compounds to capture an electron, thus triggering a chain reaction that will destroy a living cell.

Glycemic Index - Foods are ranked on a scale from 1 to 100 based on their effect on blood sugar levels.

Hypertension - High blood pressure.

Lactic acid - A colorless organic acid formed in sour milk and produced in muscle tissues during strenuous exercise.

Lipids - Fats - A class of organic compounds that are fatty acids, or their derivatives. They are not soluble in water but are soluble in organic solvents.

Macromolecules - Food broken down into usable components. A molecule containing a very large number of atoms, such as a protein or nucleic acid.

Microorganisms - A microscopic organism, such as a bacterium, virus, or fungus

Naringenin - An antioxidant, free radical scavenger, and anti-inflammatory flavanone.

Nitrosamines - Carcinogenic chemical compounds.

Nutrients - Any substance, such as protein, vitamins, or minerals that provides nourishment for the growth and maintenance of life.

Omega-3 & Omega-6 Fatty Acids - Short-chain fatty acids used to build long-chain fatty acids. The human body cannot synthesize omega fatty acids, they must be acquired through our diet.

Oxidize - The action of substances becoming combined chemically with oxygen. A chemical reaction in which electrons are lost.

Pathogenic - A bacterium, virus, or other microorganism that can cause disease.

Pectin - A soluble gelatinous polysaccharide, a carbohydrate (e.g., starch, cellulose, or glycogen) whose molecules consist of a number of sugar molecules bonded together.

pH Scale - A scale measuring from one, extremely acidic, to fourteen, extremely alkaline.

pH Balance - A balanced pH is near 7.365 on the pH scale.

Phytochemicals - The chemistry of plants and plant products.

Phytonutrients - A plant substance with nutritional value.

Protein - Essential, nitrogen-based, organic compounds of large molecules, composed of one or more long chains of amino acids.

Psoralens - Chemical compounds found in certain plants.

Purines - Metabolized chemicals that form uric acid on oxidation.

Reactants - the substances that undergo a change during a reaction.

Siddha - East Indian ancient and present-day medicine.

Soluble - Able to be dissolved, particularly in water.

Sugars - Sweet crystalline substances in plants. Soluble sweet-tasting carbohydrates such as glucose and sucrose, found in living tissues. The simple sugar glucose is an important energy source in organisms and is a component of many carbohydrates.

Toxins - Harmful chemicals.

Uric Acid - Derived from purines. When uric acid crystallizes it becomes gout.

Uricase - A digestive enzyme that breaks down purines.

Urinary Citrate - Can prevent and even cure mineral crystallization that makes kidney stones, pancreatic stones, and gallstones.

Vitamins and Minerals:

Vitamin A, Retinol - Essential for growth and vision in dim light. A yellow compound found in green and yellow vegetables and in egg yolk.

Thiamine, vitamin B1 - The first water-soluble vitamin discovered. Used in biosynthesis of gammaaminobutyric acid (GABA) and the acetylcholine. All living organisms must have thiamine, but only plants, fungi, and bacteria can synthesize it.

Riboflavin, Vitamin B2 - Riboflavin is required for metabolism of carbohydrates, proteins, fats, and ketone bodies.

Niacin, Vitamin B3 - Nicotinic Acid - Niacin contributes to DNA repair and, in the adrenal gland, the production of steroid hormones.

PantothenicAcid, vitamin B5 - A water-soluble vitamin, an essential nutrient to synthesize and metabolize carbohydrates, fats, and proteins and to synthesize coenzyme-A (CoA).

Vitamin B$_6$ - Butpyridoxal phosphate (PLP) - A cofactor in amino acid metabolism. Necessary for the enzymatic reaction in the release of glucose from glycogen.

Folate, vitamin B$_9$ - Folic Acid - Its derivatives are essential to various bodily functions, and is required to produce healthy red blood cells and prevent anemia.

Vitamin C - Supports cardiovascular health, reduces inflammation, maintains collagen, aids in growth and repair of tissue and formation of red blood cells. Humans don't synthesize ascorbate and must have it in their daily diets. Stress rapidly depletes vitamin C and the body becomes acidic.

Calcium - Calcium is central to maintaining healthy bones and in regulating the contraction of muscles.

Choline - Important in the synthesis and transport of lipids.

Copper - Found in many of the enzymes that form proteins in the body including collagen connective protein and the blood's hemoglobin.

Vitamin E - Made up of several fat soluble alcohol compounds with antioxidant properties that stabilize cell membranes.

Electrolytes - Ionized or ionizable components of blood, a cell, or other organic matter.

Iron - Essential mineral that transports oxygen throughout the body. A slight deficiency of iron causes anemia. A chronic iron deficiency can lead to organ failure.

Vitamin K - Essential for the blood-clotting process.

Magnesium - Synergistic with calcium. Magnesium ions manipulate the polyphosphate compounds of DNA, RNA, and ATP. Enzymes are dependent upon magnesium ions.

Manganese - Required trace mineral. Its enzymes are essential to detox superoxide free radicals.

Phosphorus - Essential for life, it is a component of DNA, RNA, and ATP. Cell membranes are formed of phospholipids.

Potassium - Electrolytic mineral, crucial in regulating the activity of the body's cells. Maintains proper balance of fluid in tissues and cells. Sodium and potassium produce the electrical transmissions in the nervous system, brain, and heart to keep a steady flow of electrical impulses.

Proteins - Nitrogenous organic compounds consisting of large molecules, composed of one or more long chains of amino acids.

Selenium - A trace mineral essential to good health. Incorporated into proteins to make antioxidant enzymes, selenoproteins. Some selenoproteins help prevent cellular damage from free radicals, and others build up the immune system or help regulate the thyroid.

Zinc - An essential mineral. Zinc deficiency retards growth and causes susceptibility to infections, diseases, and chronic diarrhea.

REFERENCES and RESOURCES:

https://herbs-plants.com/is-apple-cider-vinegar-anti-aging/

https://optimistminds.com/apple-cider-vinegar-to-treat-depression/

https://www.healthyandnaturalworld.com/how-to-use-apple-cider-vinegar-for-treating-arthritis/

https://medlicker.com/1235-apple-cider-vinegar-for-mycosis

https://pubmed.ncbi.nlm.nih.gov/15195908/

https://www.ncbi.nlm.nih.gov/pmc/articles/PMC5788933/#CR34

Cholesterol-lowering properties of different pectin types in mildly hypercholesterolemic men and women. *Eur J Clin Nutr*. 2012 May;66(5):591-9. doi:10.1038/ejcn.2011.208

https://curejoy.com/content/apple-cider-vinegar-for-cholesterol/

https://www.apple-cider-vinegar-benefits.com/

https://www.wikihow.com/Make-Apple-Cider-Vinegar

https://www.ncbi.nlm.nih.gov/pmc/articles/PMC4483703/

https://www.ncbi.nlm.nih.gov/books/NBK279549/

https://www.earthclinic.com/apple-cider-vinegar-for-asthma2.html

https://www.curezone.org/forums/am.asp?i=1278056

https://www.ncbi.nlm.nih.gov/pmc/articles/PMC5995450/?utm_medium=wo&utm_source=link&utm_campaign=nutrition/apple-cider-vinegar-immune-system/

https://www.wellness.guide/apple-cider-vinegar-for-cold/

https://www.ncbi.nlm.nih.gov/pmc/articles/PMC6459071/

https://howtocure.com/apple-cider-vinegar-for-ulcers/

https://adrenalfatiguesolution.com/adrenal-fatigue-symptoms/

https://diabetesjournals.org/care/article/27/1/281/26582/Vinegar-Improves-Insulin-Sensitivity-to-a-High

https://utopia.org/guide/vinegar-mother-how-to-make/

https://preserveandpickle.com/how-to-make-a-vinegar-mother/

https://well.org/nutrition/apple-cider-vinegar-immune-system-boost-or-bust/#apple-cider-vinegar-and-your-immune-system

https://pubmed.ncbi.nlm.nih.gov/29224370/

https://www.healthline.com/nutrition/6-proven-health-benefits-of-apple-cider-vinegar#4.-May-aid-weight-loss

https://scialert.net/fulltext/?doi=ijp.2016.505.513

https://www.cholesterolmenu.com/does-apple-cider-vinegar-lower-cholesterol/

https://dibesity.com/should-you-use-apple-cider-vinegar-for-weight-loss/

https://www.amazon.com/gp/product/B013J8WEEE

https://www.healthline.com/health/apple-cider-vinegar-for-colds

https://green-shack.com/apple-cider-vinegar-on-plants/

9 ways to use cider vinegar in the garden

https://www.mynoophoric.com/blogs/articles/apple-cider-vinegar-for-hair-loss-fact-or-fiction

https://www.beautyepic.com/apple-cider-vinegar-for-headache/

https://epilepsyu.com/can-apple-cider-vinegar-cure-headache/

https://www.everydayhealth.com/asthma/can-apple-cider-vinegar-help-asthma/

https://www.wellness.guide/vinegar-for-poison-oak/

https://www.ayurvedum.com/heat-exhaustion/#5-apple-cider-vinegar-treats-heat-exhaustion

https://wellnessbells.com/pneumonia/#2_Apple_Cider_Vinegar

https://www.newhealthadvisor.org/apple-cider-vinegar-for-athlete's-foot.html

https://recordrestorations.com/vd/apple-cider-vinegar-and-dizziness/

https://www.livestrong.com/article/140450-vinegar-food-poisoning/

https://herbs-plants.com/is-apple-cider-vinegar-anti-aging/

https://www.simplyandnaturally.com/eye-wash-for-cataracts/

https://easydiapering.com/apple-cider-vinegar-diaper-rash/

http://www.healthcare-online.org/Apple-Cider-Vinegar-Shingles.html

https://www.seattletimes.com/life/wellness/this-simple-hiccup-remedy-uses-apple-cider-vinegar/

https://www.verywellhealth.com/apple-cider-vinegar-and-eczema-5193751

https://stevenandersonfamily.blogspot.com/2013/11/the-cause-and-cure-of-morning-sickness.html

https://howtocure.com/apple-cider-vinegar-for-hot-flashes/

https://www.ncbi.nlm.nih.gov/pmc/articles/PMC4202636/

https://curehows.com/apple-cider-vinegar-dandruff/

https://moderncat.com/articles/apple-cider-vinegar-for-cats/

https://petkeen.com/apple-cider-vinegar-uses-benefits-for-cats/

https://www.veterinarians.org/apple-cider-vinegar-for-dogs/

https://nexusnewsfeed.com/article/health-healing/apple-cider-vinegar-can-help-prevent-obesity-1/

https://old.life-enthusiast.com/articles/apple-cider-vinegar/

https://divinitynutra.com/health/apple-cider-vinegar-neuropathy/

https://blog.nuncnu.com/can-apple-cider-vinegar-help-with-nerve-pain/

https://www.earthclinic.com/cures/sciatica.html

https://www.recipedev.com/can-apple-cider-vinegar-help-with-nerve-pain/

https://www.organicmuscle.com/blogs/organic-health-wellness/78241414-3-benefits-of-taking-apple-cider-vinegar-before-a-workout

https://www.organicmuscle.com/blogs/organic-health-wellness/78241414-3-benefits-of-taking-apple-cider-vinegar-before-a-workout

https://www.medicalnewstoday.com/articles/apple-cider-vinegar-for-colds#can-it-help

https://benefitsoffruit.com/6-brain-benefits-of-apple-cider-vinegar/

https://www.fertilitytips.com/can-apple-cider-vinegar-affect-your-fertility/

https://ndscare.com/what-does-apple-cider-vinegar-do-for-your-teeth/

https://blog.thefastingmethod.com/the-benefits-of-vinegar-hormonal-obesity-xxviii/

https://www.smartpsoriasisdiet.com/use-apple-cider-vinegar-psoriasis/

https://casachicago.org/how-to-use-apple-cider-vinegar-on-wounds/

https://www.fibromyalgiaresources.com/apple-cider-vinegar-for-fibromyalgia/

https://www.healthline.com/health/digestive-health/apple-cider-vinegar-for-constipation#use

https://www.wellness.guide/apple-cider-vinegar-for-diarrhea/

https://www.livestrong.com/article/27923-apple-cider-vinegar-remedy-asthma/

https://truedemocracyparty.net/2013/03/apple-cider-vinegar-acv-kills-cancer-anti-viral-anti-fungal-anti-bacterial-anti-septic-kills-98-of-all-germs-natures-perfect-health-food/

https://www.medicalnewstoday.com/articles/323439#what-the-research-says

https://www.beautyepic.com/apple-cider-vinegar-for-cancer/

https://www.doctorshealthpress.com/heart-health-articles/blood-pressure-articles/is-apple-cider-vinegar-good-for-high-blood-pressure/

https://natural-alternative-therapies.com/naturally-relieve-gallbladder-pain-15-minutes/

https://www.loginstep.co/

https://gallstoneclinic.com/how-does-apple-cider-vinegar-help-fatty-liver/

https://pacificpearls.com/the-health-benefits-of-eatingpearls/

https://herbs-plants.com/benefits-of-an-apple-cider-vinegar-detox-for-the-liver/

https://store.nuvisionhealthcenter.com/blogs/apple-cider-vinegar/can-apple-cider-vinegar-improve-my-digestion

https://www.recipedev.com/apple-cider-vinegar-neuropathy/

https://nashvilleveincenter.com/apple-cider-vinegar-help-varicose-veins/

https://www.verywellhealth.com/polyphenols-5217399

https://www.apple-cider-vinegar-benefits.com/vinegar-history.html

https://www.healthline.com/nutrition/6-proven-health-benefits-of-apple-cider-vinegar#:~:text=Several%20studies%20in%20animals%20and,6%2C%207%2C%208%20).

https://www.healthline.com/health/gut-health

https://www.healthline.com/health/how-to-increase-stomach-acid#:~:text=Drink%20apple%20cider%20vinegar&text=Raw%20apple%20cider%20vinegar%20can,diabetes%2C%20and%20high%20blood%20sugar

https://bmcgastroenterol.biomedcentral.com/articles/10.1186/1471-230X-7-46

https://www.ncbi.nlm.nih.gov/pmc/articles/PMC5788933/

https://www.ncbi.nlm.nih.gov/pmc/articles/PMC6453579/

https://www.ncbi.nlm.nih.gov/pmc/articles/PMC5788933/

https://www.karger.com/Article/Abstract/45180

https://pubmed.ncbi.nlm.nih.gov/19630216/

https://howtocure.com/apple-cider-vinegar-for-gout/

Thomas DeLauer:
https://www.youtube.com/watch?v=BGkpbzFda28

Thomas DeLauer
https://www.youtube.com/watch?v=vvF_w5kyyG4

https://pubmed.ncbi.nlm.nih.gov/14742438/
AMP-activated protein kinase plays a role in the control of food intake

https://pubs.acs.org/doi/abs/10.1021/jf900470c
Acetic Acid Upregulates the Expression of Genes for Fatty Acid Oxidation Enzymes in Liver To Suppress Body Fat Accumulation

https://www.ncbi.nlm.nih.gov/pmc/articles/PMC4039279/
AMPK activation—protean potential for boosting healthspan

https://pubmed.ncbi.nlm.nih.gov/29029078/
Prebiotic potential of pectin and pectic oligosaccharides to promote anti-inflammatory commensal bacteria in the human colon

https://pubmed.ncbi.nlm.nih.gov/7796781/
European Journal of Clinical Nutrition
Effect of neutralized and native vinegar on blood glucose and acetate responses to a mixed meal in healthy subjects

https://diabetesjournals.org/care/article/30/11/2814/4824/
Vinegar-Ingestion-at-Bedtime-Moderates-Waking
Vinegar Ingestion at Bedtime Moderates Waking Glucose Concentrations in Adults With Well-Controlled Type 2 Diabetes

https://www.ijmrhs.com/medical-research/effect-of-apple-cider-vinegar-on-glycemic-control-hyperlipidemia-and-control-on-body-weight-in-type-2-diabetes-patients.pdf
International Journal of Medical Research & Health Sciences: Effect of Apple Cider Vinegar on Glycemic Control, Hyperlipidemia and Control on Body Weight in Type 2 Diabetes Patients

https://blog.nuncnu.com/apple-cider-vinegar-for-kidney-stones/
Apple Cider Vinegar and Maximum Kidney & Urinary System Function

BOOKS:

The Vinegar Book
by Emily Thacker

The Apple Cider Vinegar Cure: Essential Recipes & Remedies to Heal Your Body Inside and Out
by Madeline Given, NC

81 Ways To Naturally Cleanse Your Body & House And More! The Apple Cider Vinegar Miracle
by The Alternative Daily

Apple Cider Vinegar: Nature's Most Versatile and Powerful Remedy
by Larry Jr. Trivieri

Apple Cider Vinegar for Health and Wellness: The Simple Remedy that Helps You Lose Weight, Clear Your Skin, and Boost Your Immune System
by Kathryn Young

Printed in Great Britain
by Amazon

55991855R00103